Journal of Perinatal Medicine

Vol. 16 (1988) Supplement 1

Founded by Erich Z. Saling

de Gruyter · Berlin · New York

Intrapartum Biochemical Monitoring of the Fetus

Proceedings of the First International Symposium
Atlantic City, USA, June 1987

edited by

Molly S. Chatterjee

W DE G

Walter de Gruyter
Berlin · New York 1988

Complete offprint of
Vol. 16 (1988) Supplement 1
of
Journal of Perinatal Medicine

Library of Congress Cataloging in Publication Data

Intrapartum biochemical monitoring of the fetus : proceedings of the first international
symposium, Atlantic City, USA, June 1987 / edited by Molly S. Chatterjee.
p. cm.
"Complete offprint of Vol. 16 (1988) Supplement 1 of Journal of perinatal medicine"--T. p. verso.
ISBN (invalid) 0-89925-557-6 (U.S.) : $62.00
1. Fetal blood--Analysis. 2. Transcutaneous blood gas monitoring. 3. Fetal monitoring. I. Chatterjee. Molly S., 1943- . II. Title: Biochemical monitoring of the festus.
[DNLM: 1. Blood Gas Monitoring. Transcutaneous--method-congresses. 2. Fetal Blood--analysis--congresses. 3. Fetal Monitoring--congresses. 4. Labor--congresses.
WQ 209 I6174 1987]
RG628.3.B55I58 1988
618.3'207561--dc 19 89-1714
DNLM/DLC CIP

Deutsche Bibliothek Cataloging in Publication Data

Intrapartum biochemical monitoring of the fetus :
proceedings of the ... internat. symposium. – Berlin ; New York : de Gruyter.
1. Atlantic City, USA, June 1987. – 1988
(Journal of perinatal medicine : Supplement ; Vol. 16,1)
ISBN 3-11-011586-7
NE: Journal of perinatal medicine / Supplement

 Typesetting and Printing: Gerike GmbH, Berlin. – Binding: Lüderitz & Bauer GmbH, Berlin. – Cover design: Rudolf Hübler. – Printed in Germany.

Contents

Preface

Like other developments in medicine, the monitoring of the fetus is subject to trends and fashions. After the introduction of continuous monitoring of the fetal heart rate at the end of the sixties, many obstetricians began to rely entirely on cardiotocography, neglecting fetal blood analysis which allows a much more reliable biochemical diagnosis of fetal hypoxia.

Much of what was read into cardiotographic patterns was not based on any scientific findings. This has undoubtedly inflicted discredit upon the otherwise excellent screening method. In the last few years many disappointed obstetricians have returned to a combined cardiotocographic and biochemical monitoring of the fetus during labor.

This publication should stimulate the clinicians and researchers to renew their interest in some fundamentals of biochemical monitoring.

Erich Saling, Berlin

Editor's Preface

It is my great pleasure to write this editorial for the publication of this important book on intrapartum biochemical monitoring of the fetus. A lot of hard work and difficult times have passed to materialise this publication as a supplement to the Journal of Perinatal Medicine.

This publication has been long due and without any discussion I should like to dedicate this book to the memory of my late father.

My duty as an editor of this issue will not be complete without acknowledgement of the generous contribution of Hewlett Packard and Radiometer. My personal gratitude goes to Mr. Neils Helledie, Mr. David Sands, Prof. Saling and Our Lady of Mercy Medical Center.

Molly S. Chatterjee, M.D.
Senior Fulbright Professor
New York

CIRCULATORY CHANGES AT BIRTH

Abraham M. Rudolph, Harriet S. Iwamoto, David F. Teitel

Cardiovascular Research Institute and Departments of Pediatrics and Obstetrics, Gynecology and Reproductive Sciences, University of California, San Francisco, California 94143

Introduction

Before birth, oxygenation of the fetus occurs at the placental site. Oxygenated blood is carried to the fetus through the umbilical veins; about 50% of umbilical venous blood passes through the hepatic microcirculation, but the remainder traverses the ductus venosus to the inferior vena cava (1). In the thoracic portion of the inferior vena cava, there is streaming of the well-oxygenated ductus venosus blood so that it is preferentially directed through the foramen ovale into the left atrium and left ventricle. The poorly oxygenated blood from the abdominal inferior vena cava is preferentially distributed through the tricuspid valve into the right ventricle (2, 3). This streaming pattern in the inferior vena cava, combined with the fact that almost all of the poorly oxygenated blood returning to the heart through the superior vena cava passes through the tricuspid valve, explains the presence of a higher oxygen saturation in left ventricular blood, as compared with right ventricular, in the fetus. Most of the blood ejected by the right ventricle into the pulmonary trunk bypasses the pulmonary circulation by being distributed through the ductus arteriosus directly into the descending aorta. Only a small proportion of blood ejected by the left ventricle traverses the aortic isthmus to the descending aorta, most being distributed to the head, neck, and forelimbs (4).

The foramen ovale and ductus arteriosus serve the important role of diverting blood returning to the heart away from the lungs. During fetal life, the lungs do not serve the function of gas exchange; therefore, only a small blood flow is required for metabolic functions. Were the foramen ovale not present, the total volume of fetal venous blood, including all umbilical venous as well as superior and inferior vena caval return, would have to be ejected by the right ventricle, thereby imposing a considerable unnecessary load on that ventricle. Similarly, in the absence of a ductus arteriosus, all blood ejected by the right ventricle would have to pass through the lung and return to the left ventricle, thus placing a considerable extra burden on this ventricle.

Although there is considerable streaming of umbilical venous and fetal body venous blood, the bloods do mix centrally, so that blood distributed to the fetal body as well as back to the placenta contains a mixture derived from all sources of venous return. Only a very small proportion of superior vena caval blood is, however, distributed back to the upper body.

After birth, the adult type of circulation is established, consisting of series flow of venous blood to the right atrium and ventricle, which ejects total cardiac output into the lungs, whence it returns to the left atrium and ventricle to be ejected into the aorta. There is thus no significant mixing of oxygenated arterial and poorly oxygenated venous blood. The term *cardiac output* as applied to the postnatal circulation represents the volume of blood ejected by each ventricle per minute because it refers to the volume of blood circulating in the series circuit. This concept cannot be applied in the fetus because the oxygenated and systemic venous bloods mix and are distributed both to the fetal body and to the lungs. The term *combined ventricular output* has therefore been used to designate the total volume of blood ejected by the two ventricles per minute.

To establish the adult type of circulation, several important events have to occur after birth. The umbilical-placental circulation is removed by separation of the umbilical cord, and adequate pulmonary circulation must be developed to provide oxygen to the body; also, the foramen ovale and ductus arteriosus must close. The factors responsible for effecting these changes have been examined to some extent, but separating the role of specific events that occur around birth has been difficult. Several studies were conducted in lambs exteriorized from the uterus, but with intact umbilical placental circulation (5). In similar preparations, the effects of ventilation were studied in anesthetized, open-chest lambs (6). Another approach to assessing changes after birth has been to compare measurements made in unanesthetized lambs some days after birth with those made in unanesthetized fetal lambs *in utero*. These studies have led to the current concepts that pulmonary blood flow increases markedly after birth, and that, although physical expansion of the lung alone with no change in blood gases has a small effect, the major factor responsible for the postnatal decreases in pulmonary vascular resistance is the increase in alveolar and pulmonary venous PO_2 (6). It has also been thought that elimination of the umbilical-placental circulation results in a marked increase in systemic vascular resistance, and that this is responsible for reversal of blood flow through the ductus arteriosus from the aorta to the pulmonary circulation. Furthermore, it has been thought that the main factor responsible for closure of the ductus arteriosus was the increase in aortic PO_2 (7, 8).

Measurements in newborn lambs have shown that heart rate is higher than in the fetus and that resting cardiac output (measured as the output of both ventricles to compare with the combined ventricular output of the fetus) is considerably higher (9, 10). These measurements were made two to three days after birth, so the exact time after birth that the changes occurred was not known.

Animal Model

To attempt to define the effects of some of the specific events that occur at the time of birth, we have developed a model for studying fetal lambs *in utero*. By studying the lamb within the uterus, we could avoid the interference of surface cooling and of handling, which could contribute to circulatory changes. We were able to study the effects of rhythmic ventilation alone without changing fetal blood gases, and then to examine the changes associated with oxygenation. Finally, we studied the response to occluding the umbilical cord *in utero* while the fetus was well oxygenated and ventilated. Another advantage of this preparation is that it is possible to assess the importance of some of the hormonal changes that occur immediately prior to delivery. It is well known that fetal plasma cortisol and thyroid hormone concentrations increase in the two to three days prior to birth of the lamb (11). The role of these hormonal changes on the circulatory adaptations after birth has not been well defined, although prenatal thyroid hormone is known to be important for the rise in heart rate and cardiac output after birth (12). By studying lambs before the hormonal changes have occurred and after administering selective hormones to simulate the rise that normally occurs prenatally, it will be possible to assess their importance.

We prepared 133-135 day gestation fetal lambs for study (term is ~145 days). The ewe was given epidural anesthesia and intravenous ketamine sedation. Through an abdominal incision, the uterus was exposed, and through uterine incisions over the hindlimb and over the upper left thorax, the fetus was approached. Using local anesthesia, catheters were placed in a hindlimb artery and vein. Through the fourth left intercostal space, catheters were inserted into the pulmonary trunk and left atrium and the chest closed by suturing muscle layers and skin. The head and neck were then exposed, and catheters were inserted into an external jugular vein and carotid artery. A 4.5 mm tracheal tube was passed so that its tip was in the trachea just within the thorax; it was attached to two #12 F tubes by means of a Y-connector. Through the same uterine incision, the umbilical cord was identified at the site of attachment to the abdomen, and an inflatable silicone balloon occluder was placed around it; the balloon could be inflated by injecting fluid into it through an attached catheter, resulting in umbilical vessel obstruction, which could be complete. After replacing the fetal head, the uterine incision was sutured. All catheters, including the two tracheal tubes, were led through the left maternal flank to be stored in a cloth pocket sewn to the maternal skin. The ewe and lamb were allowed to recover for two to three days; the lambs were then studied while the ewe stood quietly in a stall with access to food and water.

Fetal arterial, pulmonary arterial, left atrial, and venous pressures were measured continuously, and the heart rate, triggered from the arterial pressure pulse, was recorded beat-to-beat by means of a cardiotachometer. Blood gases and oxygen saturations were measured in each vessel during a control period and after each manipulation. Similarly, at each period combined ventricular output and its distribution as well as organ blood flows were measured by the radionuclide-labeled microsphere technique. We injected microspheres labeled with different gamma labels simultaneously into the hindlimb and left atrial catheters while blood was being withdrawn, for reference samples, from the pulmonary trunk and carotid and femoral arterial catheters. With these simultaneous injections and withdrawals, we could calculate the combined ventricular output, individual outputs of the left and right ventricles, shunts through the foramen ovale and ductus arteriosus, pulmonary blood flow, and flow to all other fetal organs and the placenta. These calculations have been described in detail (13, 14).

After making measurements during the control period, similar measurements were made during three subsequent periods:

1) The tracheal tubes were cleared of fluid and the lamb was ventilated by rhythmic expansion of the lungs with a gas consisting of about 3% oxygen and 6-7% CO_2 with the balance nitrogen. This gas mixture was chosen because the PO_2 was about 21 torr, and the PCO_2 42-49 torr, tensions similar to those in fetal blood. Using this mixture, fetal blood gases did not change significantly, so it was possible to examine the effects of rhythmic physical expansion of the lungs alone. Pressures, blood gases, and microsphere studies were measured about 15 min after the onset of ventilation.

2) Ventilation was continued, but the gas was changed to pure oxygen, with about 3-6% CO_2, sufficient to maintain fetal arterial PCO_2 constant. Again measurements were repeated about 15 min after oxygen was instituted

3) While continuing to ventilate with oxygen, the occluder on the umbilical cord was inflated to produce complete occlusion. After 15 min of occlusion, studies were repeated.

Ventilation was performed with a specially-designed respiratory pump. A continuous rapid flow of gas was maintained through the tubes during the expiratory phase to wash expired gas out of the long lengths of tubing, and thus dead space was reduced. During the inspiratory phase, positive pressures of about 25 mm Hg above amniotic cavity pressure were used. Ventilatory rates during the three phases were similar at 50 ± 9, 54 ± 10, and 56 ± 12 per min, respectively. The peak positive pressures reached during inspiration were 27 ± 10, 25 ± 10, and 25 ± 8 mm Hg above amniotic pressure during each of the three periods. Also, we found it was necessary to maintain an end-tidal pressure of 3-15 mm Hg above amniotic pressure to achieve effective lung expansion. We adjusted the inspiratory and end-expiratory pressures to achieve tidal volumes, as measured with a pneumotachograph, of 25-40 ml. The actual tidal volumes achieved during the three periods were 24 ± 15, 37 ± 16, and 31 ± 1 ml, respectively.

Effects of Rhythmic Lung Expansion

Rhythmic expansion of the lungs with the gas containing 3% oxygen produced no significant changes in fetal blood gases. Heart rate, which during the control period was 173 ± 25 per min, fell dramatically to below 100 per min with initiation of lung expansion, but within a few seconds, once rhythmic ventilation was established, it returned to a level of 152 ± 16 per min, which was slightly but not statistically significantly below control. Pressures in the aorta and pulmonary artery did not change significantly, but left atrial pressure increased from 3 ± 3 to 6.9 ± 4 mm Hg.

The combined ventricular output did not change significantly from its control value of 398 ± 81 ml/min/kg fetal weight. There was a striking increase in pulmonary blood flow from 136 ± 75 to 778 ± 513 ml/min/100 g lung weight. Pulmonary vascular resistance, calculated from mean pressure difference across the lung (mean pulmonary arterial minus left atrial mean pressure) divided by pulmonary blood flow, decreased markedly from the control value 0.44 ± 0.24 mm Hg/ml/min/100 g to 0.16 ± 0.29. There was considerable variability in the response, with some lambs showing very little change and others showing a marked fall in pulmonary vascular resistance with rhythmic lung expansion alone.

Although combined ventricular output did not change significantly, the proportions of blood ejected by each ventricle were altered. Normally in the lamb, the right ventricle ejects about two-thirds of the total output and the left, one-third (4, 13). In this series, during the control period right ventricular output was 258 ± 69 and left ventricular output 134 ± 44 ml/min/kg fetal weight, representing 66% and 34% of combined ventricular output, respectively. With lung expansion, right ventricular output fell slightly to 225 ± 69 ml/min/kg, but left ventricular output increased considerably to 211 ± 87 ml/min/kg, so that the right ventricle now contributed only 52%, whereas the left ventricle comprised 48% of combined ventricular output.

Associated with the increase in pulmonary blood flow, flows through the ductus arteriosus and foramen ovale also changed. During the control period, 57% of the combined ventricular output traversed the ductus arteriosus from the pulmonary trunk to the descending aorta and thus fell to 24% during rhythmic lung expansion; in addition, a small flow from the aorta to pulmonary artery of 3% of combined ventricular output could be calculated. Blood flow through the foramen ovale from the inferior vena cava and right atrium fell from 27% of combined ventricular output during control to 17% during lung expansion.

Blood flow to the carcass (skin, muscle, and bone) fell significantly from 15.3 ± 3.2 to 11.1 ± 4.0 ml/min/100 g tissue weight. Also, gastrointestinal blood flow fell significantly. There were also small, but not significant, changes in blood flow to the kidneys and brain, and in umbilical-placental blood flow.

Ventilation with Oxygen

Ventilation of the fetus with oxygen resulted in a marked increase of fetal arterial PO_2 from 19 ± 4 to 171 ± 164 torr. Heart rate was not significantly different from control levels. Aortic mean pressure fell from 53 ± 6 to 47 ± 6 mm Hg, and pulmonary arterial mean pressure fell from 55 ± 7 to 47 ± 6 mm Hg during oxygenation; mean left atrial pressure increased further to 8 ± 4 mm Hg.

Combined ventricular output did not change significantly from control values. Pulmonary blood flow increased even further, from 773 ± 513 ml/min/100 g lung weight during rhythmic lung expansion to 1139 ± 406 ml/min/100 g during ventilation with oxygen. Pulmonary vascular resistance fell further from the level of 0.44 ± 0.24 mm Hg/ml/min/100 g during ventilation alone to 0.04 ± 0.04 mm Hg/ml/min/100 g with oxygenation. As with rhythmic lung expansion, responses of individual lambs varied greatly. Thus, some animals showed very little pulmonary vasodilatation with lung expansion alone, but demonstrated a dramatic response with oxygenation. About half the lambs showed a major response to ventilation alone, and showed only a further small or no additional fall in pulmonary vascular resistance with oxygenation. A small number of animals demonstrated some change with ventilation and an additional similar response with oxygenation.

Associated with the increase in pulmonary blood flow, there was a further small increase in left ventricular output to 227 ± 64 ml/min/kg, whereas right ventricular output fell significantly from 225 ± 69 ml/min/kg during ventilation alone to 187 ± 47 ml/min/kg. Left ventricular output now exceeded right ventricular output with 55% of combined ventricular output being ejected by the left, and only 45% by the right, ventricle. Flow through the foramen ovale into the left atrium decreased markedly, with only 3-4% of combined ventricular output traversing the foramen. Flow through the ductus arteriosus from the pulmonary trunk to the aorta was almost completely abolished, with only about 4% of combined ventricular output flowing in this direction, but a flow of about 11% of combined ventricular output occurred from the aorta to the pulmonary arteries through the ductus arteriosus.

Blood flow to the carcass fell even further, from 11.1 ± 4 ml/min/100 g tissue during rhythmic expansion alone to 8.1 ± 3.1 ml/min/100 g during ventilation with oxygen. This represented almost 50% reduction of flow to the peripheral circulation from the control values. Cerebral flow also fell dramatically from 135 ± 53 to 58 ± 21 ml/min/100 g, and blood flow to the myocardium also fell to less than 50% of control values in association with oxygenation. Thus, left ventricular myocardial flow fell from 238 ± 126 to 102 ± 37, and right ventricular myocardial flow fell from 280 ± 97 to 113 ± 30 ml/min/100 g. A further small but insignificant fall in flow to the umbilical-placental circulation occurred.

Effects of Umbilical Cord Occlusion

The umbilical cord was occluded while the fetus was being ventilated with oxygen. No significant changes in blood gases or pH occurred as compared with ventilation with oxygen. Heart rate fell slightly in some fetuses for several seconds, but rapidly recovered so that no statistically significant changes in heart rate were noted after 15 min. Aortic pressure increased immediately with cord occlusion, and this rise was sustained, with pressure leveling at about control values. However, pulmonary arterial pressure, which dropped with oxygenation;, fell even further so that there was a significant separation of aortic and pulmonary arterial pressure. Left atrial pressure increased even more, from 8 ± 4 mm Hg during oxygenation to 10 ± 4 mm Hg after cord occlusion.

Combined ventricular output did not change significantly, and there was no further change in pulmonary blood flow or in calculated pulmonary vascular resistance. Cord occlusion resulted in no further significant change in left ventricular output, but right ventricular output did fall slightly, though not significantly. This resulted in an even greater change in the ratios of left and right ventricular outputs, with 59% of combined ventricular output now being ejected by the left ventricle. Cord occlusion resulted in no further change in right-to-left flow through the foramen ovale to the left atrium, but left-to-right shunt through the ductus arteriosus increased further slightly. Occlusion of the cord caused a significant increase in gastrointestinal blood flow from 53 ± 31 to 83 ± 34 ml/min/100 g.

Discussion

The model that we have developed permits the study of the effects of some of the individual components of the birth process on the cardiovascular adaptations after birth. It should be appreciated that although the ventilatory process we used was very effective because it was possible to maintain oxygenation and also to adequately eliminate carbon dioxide through the lungs when the umbilical circulation was abolished, it does not represent normal respiration. The positive-pressure ventilation used in this preparation could alter some of the responses that might occur with normal respiration, in which inspiration is associated with negative intrapleural pressure. In spite of this, it was possible to obtain valuable information about mechanisms involved in circulatory changes at birth.

The changes in the pulmonary circulation that we observed during each phase of our study are of particular interest. Previous studies done acutely in anesthetized open-chest exteriorized lambs by Dawes et al. (6) indicated that physical expansion of the lung with gas caused some decrease in pulmonary vascular resistance. They estimated that about one-third of the fall in pulmonary vascular resistance could be accounted for by gaseous expansion, the remainder being due to the effects of oxygen. We have confirmed these findings, except that in our studies, the effects of physical expansion of the lung, without altering blood gases, were relatively greater. What was very significant was the finding that in about half the fetal lambs studied, the increase in pulmonary blood flow, and decrease in pulmonary vascular resistance that occurred with rhythmic ventilation alone was almost maximal, and little further change resulted with oxygenation.

The mechanisms by which physical expansion decreases pulmonary vascular resistance have not been delineated. Possibly, the establishment of a gas-liquid interface at the alveolar surface tends to create a negative pressure on the small vessels, thus distending them and reducing vascular resistance. However, more recently, the possibility that lung expansion influences arachidonic acid derivatives, such as prostaglandins and leukotrienes, has been entertained. Thus, Leffler et al. (15) found that expansion of the lung in late gestation fetal lambs caused release of prostacyclin (prostaglandin I_2), which is a potent pulmonary vasodilator. It is not likely, however, that PGI_2 is completely responsible for the decrease in pulmonary vascular resistance associated with ventilation, because indomethacin, a cyclo-oxygenase inhibitor, did not prevent the fall in postnatal pulmonary vascular resistance (16), although it did modify the response. Recently, it has been suggested that leukotrienes may be implicated in perinatal pulmonary circulatory changes. Leukotriene D_4 is a potent pulmonary vasoconstrictor. Administration of either a blocker of leukotriene synthesis, or a putative leukotriene antagonist, results in a marked fall in pulmonary vascular resistance in late-gestation fetal lambs (17). The concept has been considered that the high pulmonary vascular resistance during fetal life is maintained by leukotriene action, and that the decrease after birth is related to removal of this effect. Whether lung expansion could interfere with leukotriene production is yet to be determined.

The decrease in pulmonary vascular resistance and increase in pulmonary blood flow accounts for many of the perinatal circulatory changes. Thus, the increased return of blood through pulmonary veins to the left atrium increases left atrial pressure and decreases the right-to-left flow through the foramen ovale. Also, it accounts for the reduction in right-to-left flow of blood across the ductus arteriosus, and when pulmonary vascular resistance falls markedly, there is a net left-to-right flow through the ductus. Quite apparently from these studies, elimination of the umbilical-placental circulation is not a major hemodynamic event in influencing the circulatory changes.

The increase in peripheral vascular resistance that occurred during lung expansion without oxygenation could be related to reflexes arising from the lungs. Also possibly, associated with the reduced pulmonary vascular resistance, a larger percentage of combined ventricular output is distributed to the lungs. Because combined ventricular output did not increase, the amount distributed to the fetal body falls, and the vascular resistance may increase to maintain arterial pressure.

Blood flow to the brain and the myocardium did not change with ventilation alone, but fell dramatically with oxygenation. This response is related to the profound influence that oxygen delivery has on cerebral and myocardial blood flow (18). The increase in oxygen content associated with ventilation with oxygen causes blood flow to these two organs to fall because oxygen delivery can be maintained with much lower flow rates.

Although many of the circulatory changes occurring after birth can be explained by the events examined in this study, the increase in heart rate and cardiac output was not observed. The lack of these changes could be related to many factors. We have previously shown that fetal lambs subjected to thyroidectomy about two weeks before delivery do not show the expected postnatal increase in heart rate and cardiac output (12). The lambs we studied may not have been subjected to the usual prenatal increase in thyroid hormone activity, and this could account for the lack of response. A second possible explanation is that exposure to cold may be an important factor in initiating a catecholamine response and thus producing the usual cardiovascular response. A third factor that could account for the lack of the response is that the lamb was ventilated by positive pressure. Spontaneous increase in ventilatory activity can increase heart rate in newborn lambs during hypoxemia (19), whereas fetal lambs, which do not show respiratory activity with hypoxemia, develop bradycardia (20).

In conclusion, it is apparent that the experimental model we have developed provides explanations for many of the changes in the circulation that occur during and after birth, but cannot provide mechanisms for all the changes. It will be possible, however, to examine the role of additional perinatal events, such as the effects of administration of hormones to simulate the prenatal surge in plasma hormone concentrations, and of cooling.

Acknowledgement

This research was supported by NIH grant no. HL35842.

References

(1) Edelstone DI, AM Rudolph, MA Heymann: Liver and ductus venosus blood flows in fetal lambs in utero. Circ Res 42 (1978) 426
(2) Reuss ML, AM Rudolph: Distribution and recirculation of umbilical and systemic venous blood flow in fetal lambs during hypoxia. J Develop Physiol 2 (1980) 71
(3) Edelstone DI, AM Rudolph: Preferential streaming of ductus venosus blood to the brain and heart in fetal lambs. Am J Physiol 237 (1979) H724
(4) Rudolph AM: Congenital diseases of the heart: Clinical-physiologic considerations in diagnosis and management. Year Book Medical Publishers, Chicago (1974)
(5) Assali NS, JA Morris, R Beck: Cardiovascular hemodynamics in the fetal lamb before and after lung expansion. Am J Physiol 208 (1965) 122
(6) Dawas GS: In: Foetal and neonatal physiology. Year Book, Chicago 1968
(7) McMurphy DM, MA Heymann, AM Rudolph, KL Melmon: Developmental changes in constriction of the ductus arteriosus: responses to oxygen and vasoactive substances in the isolated ductus arteriosus of the fetal lamb. Pediatr Res 6 (1972) 231
(8) Oberhansli-Weiss I, MA Heymann, AM Rudolph, KL Melmon: The pattern and mechanisms of response of the ductus arteriosus and umbilical artery to oxygen. Pediatr Res 6 (1972) 693
(9) Lister G, TK Walter, HT Versmold, PR Dallman, AM Rudolph: Oxygen delivery in lambs: Cardiovascular and hematologic development. Am J Physiol 237 (1979) H668
(10) Klopfenstein HS, AM Rudolph: Postnatal changes in the circulation, and responses to volume loading in sheep. Circ Res 42 (1978) 839
(11) Nathanielsz PW, M Silver, RS Comline: Plasma triiodothyronine concentration in the foetal and newborn lamb. J Endocrinol 58 (1973) 683
(12) Breall JA, AM Rudolph, MA Heymann: Role of thyroid hormone in postnatal circulatory and metabolic adjustments. J Clin Invest 73 (1984) 1418
(13) Heymann MA, RK Creasy, AM Rudolph: In: Proceedings of the Sir Joseph Barcroft Centenary Symposium: Foetal and neonatal physiology. Cambridge University Press, Cambridge (1973) 129
(14) Teitel DF, HS Iwamoto, AM Rudolph: Effects of birth events on central blood flow pattern. Pediatr Res 22 (1987) 557
(15) Leffler CW, JR Hessler, RS Green: The onset of breathing at birth stimulates pulmonary vascular prostacyclin synthesis. Pediatr Res 18 (1984) 938
(16) Leffler CW, TL Tyler, S Cassin: Effects of indomethacin on pulmonary vascular response to ventilation of fetal goats. Am J Physiol 234 (1978) H346
(17) Soifer SJ, RD Loitz, C Roman, MA Heymann: Leukotriene end organ antagonists increase pulmonary blood flow in fetal lambs. Am J Physiol 249 (1985) H570
(18) Peeters LLH: Blood flow to fetal organs as a function of arterial oxygen content. Am J Obstet Gynecol 135 (1979) 637
(19) Sidi D, JRG Kuipers, D Teitel, MA Heymann, AM Rudolph: Developmental changes in oxygenation and circulatory responses to hypoxemia in lambs. Am J Physiol 245 (1983) H674
(20) Cohn HE, EJ Sacks, MA Heymann, AM Rudolph: Cardiovascular responses to hypoxemia and acidemia in fetal lambs. Am J Obstet Gynecol 120 (1974) 817

INTRODUCTION AND CLINICAL ASPECTS OF BIOCHEMICAL MONITORING OF THE FETUS

Erich Saling

Institute of Perinatal Medicine of the Free University of Berlin, Mariendorfer Weg 28, D-1000 Berlin 44, Germany

General Introduction

Biochemical monitoring of the fetus during labor seen from the aspect of medical history as a whole is like an infant just born. But when considering it within the 25 year age of perinatal medicine it is like a steam engine of old generation. Its maiden voyage - the first fetal blood analysis - took place on 21st June 1960 (36).

Modern, safe supervision of the fetus during labor involves two methods:

1. Cardiotocography as a way of continuous electronic monitoring of the fetus to detect early signs of threatened hypoxia.
2. A biochemical method - at the present time, fetal blood analysis, which should only be employed as a complementary measure in cases with suspicious or pathological cardiotocogram.

An additional biochemical method enables us:

a. to clarify whether or not biochemical changes confirm imminent fetal hypoxia and/or acidosis which has been indicated by cardiotocography; and
b. to help in deciding whether further important clinical consequences like tocolysis for inhibition of uterine contractions or termination of labor by operation are necessary. In this way by using both cardiotocography and if

necessary additionally fetal blood analysis, it is possible to achieve a minimum of operative deliveries which is of advantage to the mothers, with an optimum of safety for the fetus.

From our many years of experience and in my own personal view, the consistent additional use of fetal blood analysis could have avoided some of the problems and criticisms which occurred in several countries during the past in connection with the sole use of cardiotocographic supervision during labor and the increased cesarean section rate.

Pathophysiology of fetal hypoxia during labor and consequences on the state of the newborn

Hypoxia leads primarily to an initial decrease in the pH values in the blood caused by the accumulation of CO_2 and thus to respiratory acidosis; this would be stage I in the illustratively demonstrated step-by-step development of hypoxia and acidosis (Fig. 1).
Secondly in stage II there is an additional overloading of organic acids, leading to combined acidosis. Due to anaerobic glycolysis this mainly concerns the lactic acid; the blood pH levels decrease still further.
In the third phase, in stage III the acidosis which has progressed in the meantime, and which is predominantly of metabolic character, begins to have a negative effect on the whole organism. The central nervous system becomes depressed and so - depending on the duration - incisive changes occur, having a depressing effect on the muscles, the reflexes, the respiration and the circulation. If the infant is born during this stage - that is stage III - reduced Apgar Score can often certainly be expected.

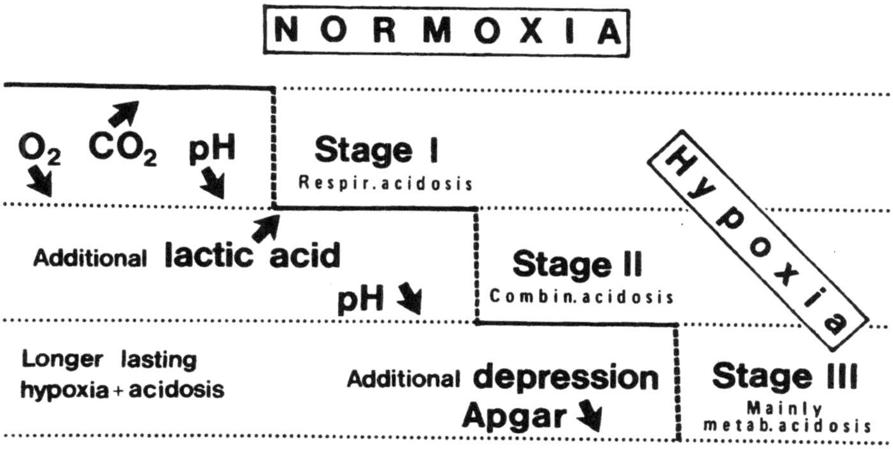

Figure 1

If other depressive influences play an additional role apart from the hypoxic causes described here, for example due to previous application of pain relieving drugs or anesthesia, then of course the Apgar Score can deteriorate earlier on.

The characteristics and clinical importance of these three pathophysiological stages are often being misunderstood. Situations occurring during labor are described for example a pathological CTG or even decreasing fetal pH-values, which are afterwards compared with the Apgar-Score. "False positive" findings during labor are said to have been present in infants where the Apgar-Score was "still" good. Bearing in mind what has already been said, it must be clear how naive this scientifically untenable conclusion is. Neither a pathological CTG caused by hypoxia nor decreasing pH-levels lead immediately - that is from the very beginning - to a reduced Apgar-Score. An appropriate long latency period must

be taken into consideration. If an infant is born before Stage III it will often still be vigorous. This is certainly not a "false positive" finding - from the clinical aspect - but rather a "correct positive" one.
To assess the state of the newborn only by using the Apgar-Score is antiquated and inadequate. This is why the state of the newborn should never be assessed by this method alone. Much better post partum hypoxia diagnostics in the newborn can be achieved by using a combination of the Apgar-Score and measurements of the pH in the umbilical cord blood, which we introduced into clinical routine practice in 1965 (27).

Suitability of fetal blood samples

As long ago as 1966 Desai et al. (11) reported a good correlation between pH blood gas values in samples taken from the newborn scalp and from a branch of the temporal artery so that they recommended scalp samples for monitoring newborn. Later Adamsons et al. (1) showed that there was an excellent correlation in experimental animals between blood samples from the scalp and from the carotid or jugular arteries. Between 1964 and 1970, Bowe et al. (6), Gare et al. (13), Kubli et al. (18), Teramo (37) and ourselves (5) all found that there was a good correlation during labor between values in human fetal blood samples and those in the umbilical vessels. O'Connor et al. (22) published - as far as FBA is concerned - a dissenting view. However later on several comments from various authors, namely Furi and Beard (12), Philip (23), Rooth et al.(25), including a contribution from ourselves (34) have disproved these statements. Our publication of 1976 (5) apparently unknown to O'Connor et al. pointed out that even in cases of moderate or marked caput succedaneum the correlation between the pH of scalp and of umbilical arterial blood was surprisingly good. Concerning actual pH, r was 0.78 and for pH after equilibration, r was 0.79.

What do fetal scalp blood samples express?

We analyse microblood samples from the peripheral circulation. The composition does not differ too much from arterial blood, because the arterio-venous difference in the peripheral circulation is estimated as being relatively small on account of the low metabolism in the skin. There is no difference in the composition of the blood between arteries to the brain and those supplying the scalp, as they both receive blood from the same main branches of the aorta. Of course, it would be more informative to analyse venous blood from those organs of special interest, for instance from the brain. However, this is up to now scarcely possible in routine clinical work. However, for diagnostic purposes it is important to know that particularly in chronic hypoxia the fetus undergoes the so-called O_2 conserving adaptation of its circulation (31) and as a result of this pathophysiological mechanism the supply to the brain and heart is affected much later; other organs such as the skin, muscles and intestines are subjected to a reduced O_2 supply much earlier.
Recent results from simultaneous Doppler ultrasound investigations in the fetal common carotid artery and the fetal aorta achieved by ARABIN et al. in our institute (2) provide an interesting new confirmation of the O_2 conserving adaptation concept. In severely growth retarded fetuses ratio of blood flow volume of the common carotid artery to the fetal aorta was significantly increased.
It is also known from the pathophysiology of the cerebral circulation, that even in cases of significant changes of

blood pressure in the body circulation, a stable supply of blood to the brain is maintained, through the highly adjustable autoregulation of the brain circulation (19). Accordingly, we can assume that generally before the brain circulation is affected there will have been disturbances in the periphery, for instance in the muscles, leading to anaerobic glycolysis and to the overproduction of lactic acid. Thus, through fetal blood analysis and the falling pH values or increasing $tcPco_2$ values we get warning signs early enough, and can draw the necessary conclusions. Most of these considerations also concern the conditions using transcutaneous blood gas measurements.

It is rather doubtful whether - as Mann and coworkers (20) found - an isolated severe cerebral ischemia can occur with substantial head compression accompained by bradycardia, with subsequent permanent psycho-motor impairment of the infant. Follow-up examinations of children with increased intracranial pressure showed a higher incidence of abnormalities only after more than 20 hours of protracted labor (21). From these results it can be concluded that relatively short lasting head compression does not seem to be seriously dangerous.

We recently found in a prospective study performed together with Maria Brand concerning intracranial hemorrhage, that in cases with fetal bradycardia and/or variable decelerations in the cardiotocogram without an accompanying hypoxia (this means with normal pH-values), there was no higher incidence of cases with brain hemorrhage (7a, 7b). It is known that particularly hemodynamic factors are main causes of brain hemorrhage.

Suitable biochemical parameters for the clinical supervision of the fetus

For purely clinical purposes it is sufficient to perform only blood pH measurements. Direct blood gas measurements can be dispensed with, since simultaneously with the occurrence of hypoxemia, there is also a CO_2 increase which leads to a fall of pH-values and thus to a respiratory acidosis. Later an O_2 insufficiency leads to an increase of lactic acid content and to a metabolic acidosis of the infant through anaerobic glycolysis. Both kinds of increases in acidity can be ascertained by measurements of the falling pH-values. The growing possibility of continuous transcutaneous measurements in the fetus can provide interesting additional information; particularly the $tcPco_2$ measurements which will be reported later at this symposium by Dr. Schmidt who elaborated interesting results in our unit.

Non hypoxic acidity increase in the fetus

There is one possibility which should be excluded namely the so-called maternogenic increase of fetal acidity. This situation is caused by overflow of lactic acid from the mother to the fetus. To rule out such cases with maternogenic origin of acidity increase we recommend to measure maternal and fetal acidity and to compare either the actual pH-values which has been recommended by Rooth et al. (24) or the pH-values of metabolic acidity, which has been recommended by us (26). The latter means the pH after equilibration of the blood sample with 40 mmHg of Pco_2. We call this pH abbreviated pHqu40.

Such maternogenic increased acidity plays a clinical role in only about 10% in all cases with acidosis (Fig. 2) and only less than 1% in cases with more serious acidosis of less than 7.10 pH (14). If the difference between mother and fetus is less than 0.15 between the actual pH values or the difference of pHqu40 is less than 0.05, maternogenic acidity increase is confirmed. Such a situation is not as dangerous as acidosis caused by fetal hypoxia. Therefore it is not necessary to terminate the labor immediately by operation. An operative intervention would only be recommendable if pH decreases to slight acidotic values.

	No acidosis	Acidosis			
UApH act / Type of acidity increase	7.29–7.20 (n = 590)	≤ 7.19 (n = 268)	≤ 7.09 (n = 77)	≤ 6.99 (n = 20)	Σ (n = 858)
FAI_{S+R}	244 (52%)	226 (48%)	75 (16%)	20 (4%)	470 (100%)
MAI_{S+R}	346 (89%)	42 (11%) $p < 0.0001$	2 (0.5%) $p < 0.0001$	– $p < 0.04$	388 (100%)
FAI_S	359 (60%)	238 (40%)	76 (13%)	20 (3%)	597 (100%)
MAI_S	231 (89%)	30 (11%) $p < 0.0001$	1 (0.5%) $p < 0.0001$	– $p < 0.04$	261 (100%)
FAI_R	347 (59%)	244 (41%)	75 (13%)	20 (3%)	591 (100%)
MAI_R	243 (91%)	24 (9%) $p < 0.0001$	2 (1%) $p < 0.0001$	– $p < 0.04$	267 (100%)

Subdivision of the FAI and MAI newborns depending on their UApH-act values and the differently defined acidity increases

FAI = fetogenic acidity increase

MAI = maternogenic acidity increase

R = after ROOTH (M/F Δ $pH_{akt} \leq 0.15$)

S = after SALING (M/F Δ $pH_{qu40} \leq 0.05$)

Figure 2

Clinical benefits of additional biochemical monitoring

a) Advantages and disadvantages of cardiotocography

The controversies about intensive monitoring of the fetus during labor have arisen from the very beginning - that is since cardiotocography was first introduced into clinical routine practice in 1968. Two of the important questions to do with the suitability of this method were not properly differentiated from each other, namely:

1. with what reliability do suspicious or pathological heart rate patterns occur when fetal hypoxia and acidosis are really present (Fig. 3 upper part) and
2. how often is fetal hypoxia really present, when suspicious or pathological heart rate patterns occur in the cardiotocogram (lower part).

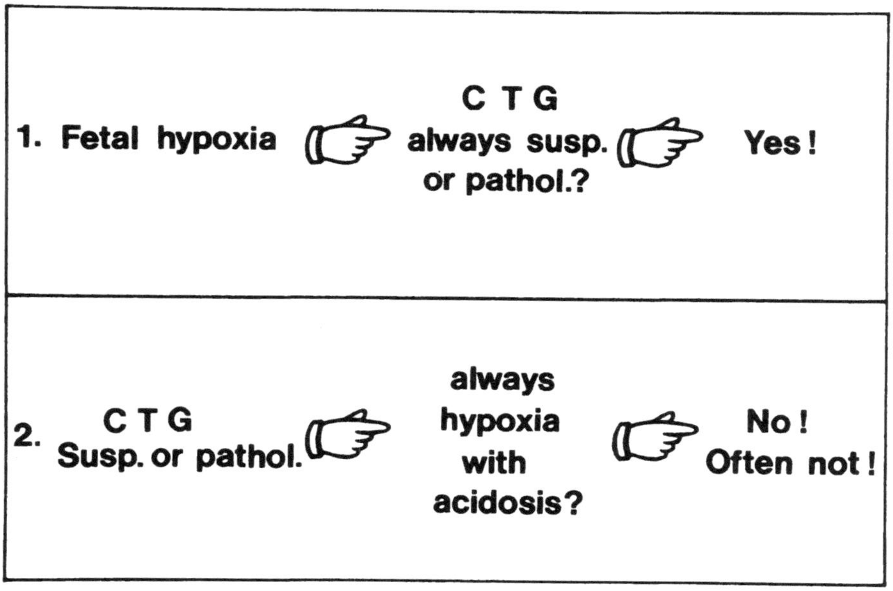

Figure 3

As regards the first point, cardiotocography is an excellent and reliable method, because one can be certain that almost all fetal hypoxias will be detected early enough by the occurrence of any abnormal heart rate pattern. This has however unfortunately led to the ill-fated erroneous assumption that there is an equally high reliability as far as the second question is concerned,- that is that suspicious or pathological heart rate patterns are always an expression of fetal hypoxia. This is definitely not the case for hypoxia and acidosis are often not imminent or present when suspicious or pathological heart rate patterns occur on the cardiotocogram. At the end of the sixties and beginning of the seventies (28, 29, 30, 32) we pointed out very clearly that cardiotocography was unreliable in providing correct evidence of threatened or existing hypoxia and acidosis. Even when all pathological heart rate patterns are present in such a severe form the cardiotocographic diagnosis can still be incorrect. We published such a record as far back as 1973 (33).

b) Our more recent results concerning cardiotocography and fetal pH-values

A more recent evaluation in our unit, drawn up together with Goeschen and Gruner, provides interesting results (15). 407 patients were continuously monitored by cardiotocography during labour and if suspicious or pathological heart rate patterns occurred were additionally monitored by fetal blood analysis. The cardiotocogram was assessed using the complicated, but still most reliable procedure, namely the Hammacher-Score (16). As far as cardiotocography can be exactly evaluated at all under strong scientific conditions, the Hammacher-Score is still the most objective procedure because all the three assessment criteria - the baseline fetal heart rate, the contraction related fetal heart rate, (the so called decelerations) and the variability of the baseline (the so called fluctuations or oscillations) - the latter even with their number and with the amplitude - are included in this score. From our point of view a more objective assessment of a cardiotocogram does not exist.

Firstly it could be seen in our evaluations that (Fig. 4) also according to the Hammacher-Score in 80% of these cases the CTG could be regarded as abnormal; 3 or more points were present. In 78% of these suspicious or pathological cases (right part) the pH values of the fetus obtained by fetal blood analysis were optimal, that is 7.30 and better; in 12% they were slightly reduced but still within the normal range - that is between 7.29 and 7.25. Taken as a whole therefore, normal pH values were measured in 90% of these fetuses and prepathological or pathological values (pH below 7.25) in only 10%.

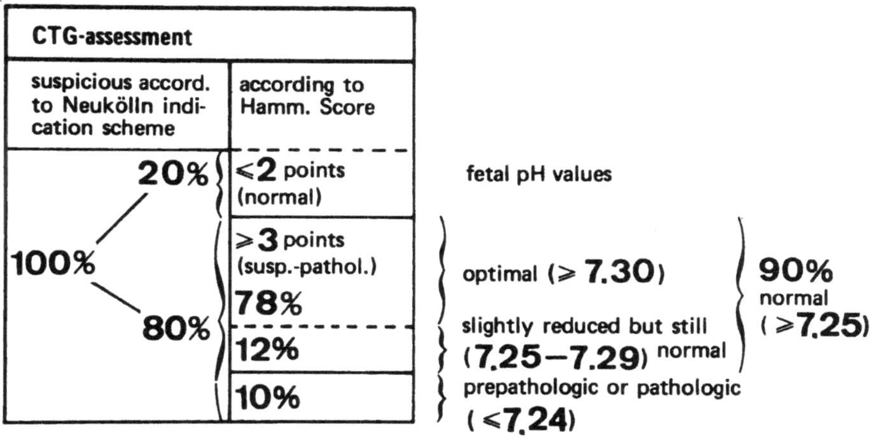

Figure 4

As was to be expected, the number of cases with reduced pH values increased as the CTG score deteriorated (Fig. 5). However it cannot be said that this would allow reliable clinical conclusions to be drawn. Even with prepathological and pathological CTG scores with 5 points and more the number of cases with preacidosis or acidosis only amounted to 26%.

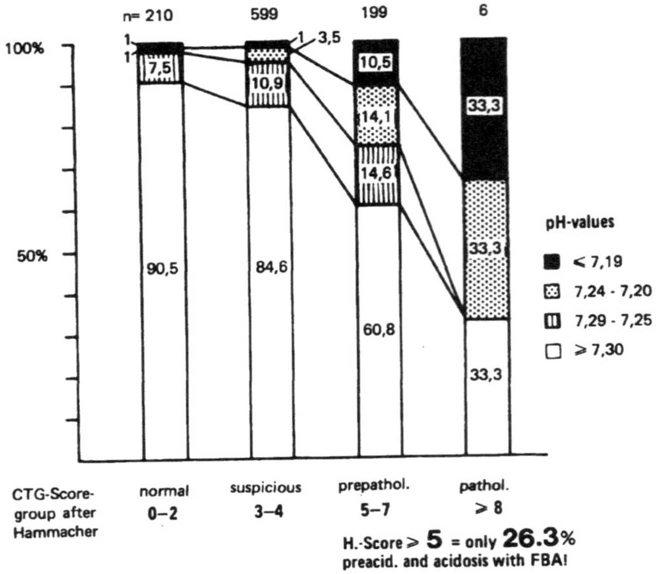

Figure 5

If, not having used fetal blood analysis, we had regarded an operative termination of the labour as indicated from 4 Hammacher Score points onwards - which is a logical clinical consideration - operative interventions would have been necessary in 73% of these risk cases concerned (Fig. 6) in order not to miss the 14% of fetuses who really were at high risk due to a fall in pH values. So here we have an over-diagnosis through cardiotocography of around 60%.

When using fetal blood analysis the following clinical results in all our cases were achieved: in 46% of the cases the delivery was spontaneous and in 54% operative. If the first stage and the second stage are subdivided, the following picture emerges:

in the first stage an operative delivery - mostly a cesarean section due to suspicious or pathological cardiotocogram - would have been indicated in 56% of the cases. After

performing fetal blood analysis, however, the cesearan section rate was only 10% - this means a saving of 46%.
Also in the second stage decisive advantages were found when combined monitoring was used. Here a CTG score of ≥4 was recorded in 95% of the cases. Instead of having to operate on all these high risk cases, through the results achieved by fetal blood analysis, it was only really necessary to make an operative intervention in 54% of them. The remaining 41% infants could be delivered spontaneously.

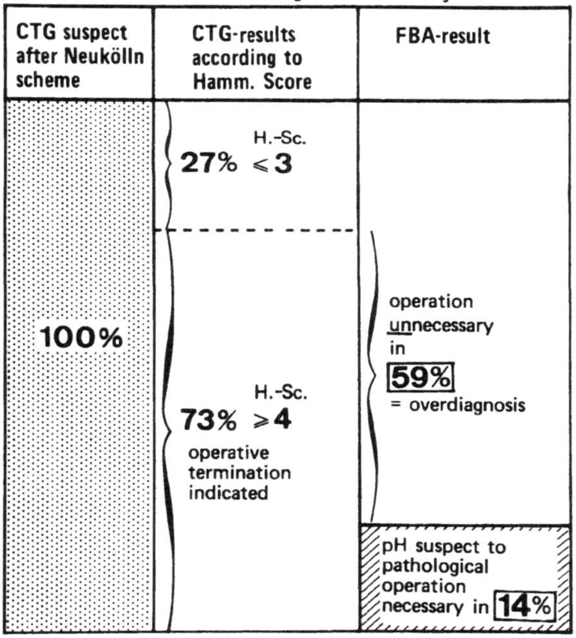

Figure 6

According to our experience fetal blood analysis is indicated in the early second stage, when the cervix is completely dilated but the presenting part is still in the pelvic inlet or in the mid-pelvic plane. When the presenting part is already in the pelvic floor or pelvic outlet (late second stage) and suspicious or pathological patterns occur in the cardiotocogram the labor is terminated immediately without fetal blood analysis. In this case the operative intervention is fairly simple and therefore no advantage would be gained by awaiting the results of fetal blood analysis.

Operative interventions in the early second stage (vacuum extractions) - that is from the pelvic inlet or the mid-pelvic plane - can by no means be regarded as harmless for the fetus. Often they require difficult manipulation and should therefore only be performed when there is a strong clinical indication, and never without such a strong reason, for example when the CTG patterns are suspicious or pathological not due to hypoxia. In the already mentioned prospective study (7a,7b) we were able to show (Fig. 7) that intracranial hemorrhage (mostly slight) occurs twice as frequently in mature infants delivered operatively in the early second stage (10.5%) than in the late second stage (4.5%) and almost four times more frequently than in infants delivered spontaneously (2.6%).

Vaginal operative deliveries and ICH

according to SALING and BRAND

n = 218 ICH = 18 = 8.3%

	Mature inf. (> 37/0)			Premature inf. (< 37/0)		
	total n	ICH n	ICH %	total n	ICH n	ICH %
Pelvic inlet	30	2	6.7	1	0	(0)
Mid-pelvic plane	75	9	12.0	5	1	(20.0)
Early 2nd stage	105	11	10.5	6	1	(16.7)
Mid-pelvic plane – pelvic floor	37	2	5.4	7	1	(14.3)
Pelvic floor+ pelvic outlet	52	2	3.8	11	1	(9.1)
Late 2nd stage	89	4	4.5	18	2	(11.1)
Σ	194	15	7.7	24	3	(12.5)
Spontaneous delivery	801	21	2.6	87	19	21.8

Figure 7

At the 11th German Congress of Perinatal Medicine (35) in November 1983 we tried to give a less scientific but impressive and illustrative description of the advantages and disadvantages of cardiotocography in simple terms. For this purpose we took an example from nature. The cardiotocogram situation can be compared with the screaming of monkeys in the jungle: when danger is imminent they always scream. When there is a threat of hypoxia, the CTG is almost always suspicious or pathological. But monkeys have the typical attribute of screaming much too often; especially when there is no danger at all. The CTG often does this too, in the figurative sense. It is suspicious or pathological, but there are no real reasons to suspect dangerous fetal hypoxia - as measurements of the acid-base balance can clearly prove. This is unfortunately the reverse side of cardiotocography which many obstetricians either fail to recognize or push aside with naive credulity. If the newborn are vigorous after operative delivery - as regards their acidity and clinical state - then many colleagues excuse their management by saying that a hypoxia had just been avoided by well-timed intervention. Anyone who performs fetal blood analysis or even transcutaneous Pco_2 measurements, can give enough examples how often such excuses are self deception or a misguidance to the patient.

There has been so much speculation and so many hypotheses mixed with physiological and pathophysiological facts concerning the regular circle of heart rate behavioural patterns, that as far as daily clinical requirements are concerned reality is overlooked.

I assume internal specialists or anesthetists would laugh at us if we wanted to suggest in all seriousness, that it is possible to draw definite conclusions in adults as to whether the patient concerned was suffering from hypoxia or not merely by the interpretation of the heart rate patterns alone. This suggestion must appear to be even more curious, since biochemical methods of measuring parameters in the blood gases and in acid-base balance have already been in existence for 25 years and provide a much more reliable diagnosis of hypoxia, namely a direct one. Unfounded arguments are used in the debate that fetal blood analysis is too complicated and too expensive. These ignore the high costs of staff, material and treatment caused by the numerous cesarean sections performed unnecessarily, and also the negative consequences of complications that often occur after such operations.

Comment on some publications concerning basic questions of biochemical monitoring

Modern intensive monitoring of the fetus during labor - and in particular biochemical monitoring - have sometimes been the subject of dubious criticism and arguments. The unshakeable belief in prospective studies can impair the judgement for clinical reality. For example HAVERCAMP et al. (17) have made comparisons between auscultatory, cardiotocographical and also cardiotocographical and biochemical monitoring in groups that were much too small. They also overlooked the fact that a purely auscultatory monitoring is not practised over a long period of time anywhere in the world under the same conditions as for such a prospective model study. The question has to be asked what is the practical clinical benefit of such studies at all. Furthermore in the few cases where intrauterine complications did in fact occur, the authors only then took the necessary action when acidoses had already occurred. It is not surprising that results were then achieved which did not show any differences between the compared methods.
These results which we think are misleading have been quoted a lot and have caused much confusion. When comparing the results of Havercamp and coworkers with our retrospectively evaluated material under the same group divisions, much worse

results were to be found in the Havercamp study (Fig. 8).

		total No.	patho-logical	%	significant difference
UApH≤7.20	Havercamp et al.	212	38	17.9	
	Our high risk cases FBA–group	1333	182	13.7	no
	Our total material 1978 + 1979 *	4720	437	9.3	yes, p:0.04
Apgar Score≤7 **1min**	Havercamp et al.	230	73	31.7	
	Our high risk cases FBA–group	1333	119	8.9	yes, $p < 0.001$
	Our total material 1978 + 1979 *	4649	282	6.1	yes, $p < 0.001$
Apgar Score≤7 **5min**	Havercamp et al.	230	12	5.2	
	Our high risk cases FBA–group	1330	22	2.9	no
	Our total material 1978 +1979 *	4350	75	2.7	yes, p: 0.02

* The total material from our department consistently includes a high percentage of cases with risk factors (in 1970 the rate amounted to 80.8%)

Figure 8

For example the number of "acidoses" in the umbilical artery blood at 18% was twice as frequent and significantly higher in the Havercamp group, compared to 9% in our group. Our total material contains a high percentage of risk cases. The difference in the 1 minute Apgar-Score is even more striking. The number of depressed infants amounted to 32% in the Havercamp group, and in our group it was only 6%. Even if we compare the Havercamp results with our highest risk group in which all cases had a pathological cardiotocogram and therefore fetal blood analyses were performed, the frequency of depressed infants (1 minute Apgar-Score 7 and less) was 9% in our group and 32% in the Havercamp group. Also our incidence of cases with "acidosis" was lower but not significantly. However, since - according to strict theoretical conceptions - apparently only prospective studies provide truthful results, such a comparison is open to attack.

We do agree with Havercamp on one point, that intensive monitoring during labor done in an unskilled fashion - particularly when cardiotocography is used exclusively - leads to an unnecessarily high rate of cesarean sections and other operative deliveries. Particularly this topic has been recently discussed in our publication together with van den BERG and S.SCHMIDT in the British Journal of Obstetrics and Gynaecology (4).

CLARKE and PAUL theorized in a publication in 1985 (10) and argued amongst other things, that in 25 perinatal centers in the United States fetal blood analysis had been performed on only about 3% of the parturients. They list six reasons for practical problems and thus explain why fetal blood analysis is not more widespread. According to our experience most of the reasons are of little or no importance. On the other hand, there were objections like unavailability of technical personell and equipment, technical difficulty in performing the procedure, time delay in obtaining results, misinterpretation of data, insufficient initial training. These problems would also seriously jeopardize any other medical procedure, if one were not able to solve such basic but typical difficulties of poor organisation, inexperience or prejudice. An objective observer will not be convinced by such a weak line of argument.

In our unit with about 3,000 deliveries per year and around 20% of cases with fetal blood analyses, none of the reasons mentioned above creates an essential practical problem which would make performing fetal blood analysis an unreasonably expensive or difficult procedure. In my opinion the authors of such publications - in the interest of an objective investigation should previously have visited the place where fetal blood analysis was developed and where - as in no other center - practical and clinical experience has been collected in the meantime on more than 17,000 cases, and should then check on the real reasons why there are so different opinions on biochemical monitoring.

Further, Clark and Paul (10) made some other statements, namely "... an acidotic scalp blood pH (< 7.20) was associated with an Apgar-Score of 7 and more, that is a false prediction of fetal compromise ... Another comment: "in recent large series it has been reported that 73% of infants with an umbilical arterial pH of less than 7.10, a level usually viewed as indicative for severe fetal acidosis, nevertheless had a one minute Apgar score of 7 and more. In 86% of these infants the five minute Apgar score was more than 7". They draw the following conclusions from this statement: "such data raise serious questions about the actual superiority of fetal blood pH measurement over fetal heart rate assessment in the prediction of fetal compromise." Concerning all these comments they overlook the fact that the consequences of intrauterine hypoxia have a step-by-step course as we have already clearly explained, and therefore the results which they find surprising are - pathophysiologically seen - apparently logical.
Many other examiners make the same mistake by comparing the results of biochemical monitoring during labor with Apgar Score and often also with umbilical pH values. They are then disappointed to find that there are so many so called "false positive" findings. Those authors believe as if it would be clinically inevitable for a newborn infant to be depressed or acidotic when suspicious or decreasing pH values have been present during labor. Also a deception lies in the fact that in addition to the pathophysiological facts mentioned above, the real clinical situation is not given enough consideration. Surely the aim of modern obstetrics is to deliver - if only possible - a clinically vigorous infant even after the first manifest signs of the beginning of intrauterine hypoxia have been detected, for example when the pH values have apparently fallen or transcutaneously measured Pco_2 levels have apparently increased, both in spite of the administration of tocolytic drugs.

If labor is in the first stage, then the obstetrician must also assess the latency period from the moment of the diagnosis to the probable time of the delivery by cesarean section. The decision-delivery time, which generally lasts from about 7 to 15 minutes in emergency cases, must be taken into consideration. In some cases the pH-values will improve up to the operative delivery of the infant, if the complications are of a transitory character. The number of such cases is however rather small. In the majority of the cases with confirmed progressive increase of acidity, the pH values drop to the prepathological range (7.24 - 7.20), sometimes even to the pathological range (< 7.20). If in such cases the fetus is delivered by operative intervention fast enough, then most of the newborn will have a normal Apgar Score (Fig. 9) as is to be expected after the step-by-step course of hypoxia described above. Therefore we should value the Apgar Score as a reference parameter in these studies with more caution. It is

Typical example for erroneously so called „wrong positive" result

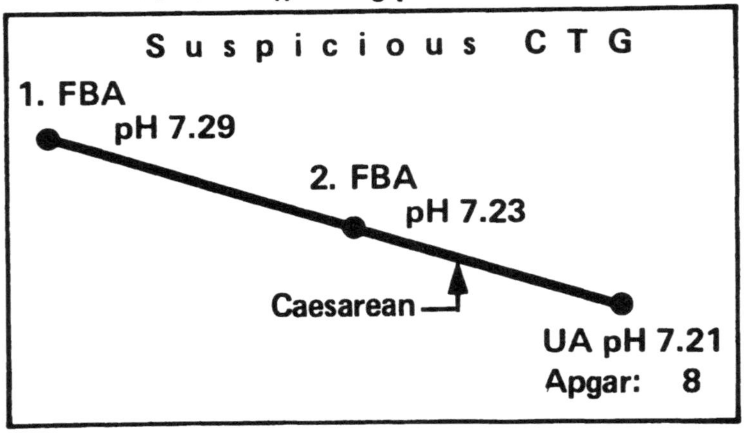

Operative delivery indicated by real fetal distress
CTG=Cardiotocogram, FBA=Fetal blood analysis

Figure 9

much more reliable to compare the findings of an acidity increase in the fetus with the pH levels in the umbilical artery blood.

After taking all these points into consideration, an equally high or even only slightly decreased pH level in the umbilical artery blood (Fig. 9) is an argument for a correct positive diagnosis and not - as is often maintained after incorrect observations - for a false positive one.

We should bear in mind that the prime concern is to find out how far a method of supervision fulfils the task which we expect from it. In this way too a great amount of confusion in the clinical observations on supposedly so frequent false positive findings could have been avoided.

We are just performing such a study together with Sabine Brand and P. van den Berg (8). Out of 110 fetuses (Fig. 10) which

"Correct" and "false" positive cases monitored by FBA

Operative delivery because of reduced FBA pH-values (< 7.25)		n = 110 = 100 %		
Umb.-art. pH	< 7.20	n = 62 = 56.4%	93.6%	"Correct" positive
Umb.-art. pH	7.20–7.24	n = 41 = 37.3%		
Umb.-art. pH	⩾ 7.25	n = 7 =	6.4%	"False" positive

After S. Brand, P. van den Berg, E. Saling

Figure 10

had an abnormal cardiotocogram and simultaneously reduced scalp pH-values (< 7.25), 94% had an equal or lower pH-value in umbilical artery samples. Only 6.4% had higher pH-values, this means that fetal blood analyses have been misleading and in so far are really "false positive".On the other hand only 4 newborns, that is 3.6%, have been severely depressed with an Apgar Score of 2 or less. As we have already pointed out in our comparison with the HAMMACHER-Score, cardiotocography for clinical purposes leads much too frequently to false diagnoses.

Clarke et al. made a good suggestion by introducing the fetal scalp stimulation in order to save a number of fetal blood analyses (9).

To a large extent we agree with the much discussed publications of Banta and Thacker (3) on the question of electronic fetal monitoring, that cardiotocography leads to a high rate of unnecessary cesarean sections, and that as a result there is an increase in maternal morbidity and mortality that could have been avoided.

When considering such aspects I am surprised to see that on the one hand American lawyers are very active in charging obstetricians when they have made a supposed or genuine mistake with regard to the impairment of the infant. On the other hand American lawyers have not yet realised what they could make by charging another kind of malpractice, - namely, that numerous avoidable impairment occurs particularly through maternal morbidity - because no high quality diagnoses is performed to avoid unnecessary cesarean sections. The mere thought of this prospect should inspire those colleagues who often operate unnecessarily, to perform better obstetrics.

We disagree with several conclusions of Banta and Thacker because - as previously described in detail - both these authors rely on the scientifically untenable assessment of the sensitivity of biochemical monitoring on account of the so called false positive results discussed several times in this presentation. Unfortunately therefore the basis of the many essential considerations in this otherwise well constructed and commendable study is lost to a high degree.

General review of intensive supervision during labor

The use of intensive supervision of the fetus during labor should also be regarded from a more superordinated point of view. We know that the birth process - even when uncomplicated - is a relatively short period of concentrated occurrences, which nowadays take their course within, lets say, less than 18 hours. In no other period of our life are we threatened by such concentrated risks in such a short space of time. It is also apparent that we recognize labor by the well known symptomes, like the start of contractions with or without the membranes having ruptured, and are thus able to recognize the beginning of the birth process. As a rule labor is not included among the unforeseeable events that happen unexpectedly, as for example is often the case with a heart attack. To know that moments of considerable danger are concentrated within a few certain hours of our life, and nevertheless to renounce on intensive supervision for such a period of time, is in my eyes reckless.

Final Remarks

In conclusion it should be said: combined cardiotocographical and biochemical supervision is inseparable and offers the highest possible safety concerning complications caused by hypoxia. Numerous observations in the literature show how often medicine is susceptible to subjective interpretations, pseudo argumentation and arbitrary statements.
I strongly recommend anyone who has still not been convinced by my arguments, to get acquainted with continuous transcutaneous blood gas measurements on the fetus,

particularly $tcPco_2$ registrations if he is not experienced with fetal blood analysis. I am in no doubt whatsoever, that the person concerned will then recognize at the latest the high clinical value of additional biochemical monitoring and also what was lacking in the past.

References

(1) Adamsons K, RW Beard, RE Myers: Am J Obstet Gynecol 107 (1970) 435

(2) Arabin B, PL Bergmann, E Saling: Fetal Therapy (in press)

(3) Banta HD, SB Thacker: Obstet Gynec Surv 34 (1979) Suppl 627

(4) van den Berg P, S Schmidt, J Gesche, E Saling: Br Obstet Gynaec 94 (1987) 72

(5) Boenisch H, E Saling: J Perinat Med 4 (1976) 45

(6) Bowe ET, RW Beard, M Finster, PJ Popper, K Adamsons, LS James: Am J Obstet Gynecol 107 (1970) 279

(7a) Brand M, E Saling: Arch Gynecol 238 (1985) 263

(7b) Brand M, E Saling: In: Kubli F: Perinatal Brain Damage. Springer, Heidelberg 1988

(8) Brandt S, P van den Berg, E Saling: The significance of so called "false positive" results in monitoring of the fetus during labor. (in preparation)

(9) Clark SL, ML Gimovsky, C Miller: Am J Obstet Gynecol 148 (1984) 274

(10) Clark SL, RH Paul: Am J Obstet Gynecol 153 (1985) 717

(11) Desai SD, R Holloway, AK Thambiram: Lancet (1965) 1126

(12) Furi L, RW Beard: Lancet I (1980) 483

(13) Gare DJ, CG Whetham, JD Henry: Am J Obstet Gynecol 99 (1967) 722

(14) Goeschen K, R Höhn, JW Dudenhausen, E Saling: Z Geburtsh u Perinat 188 (1984) 68

(15) Goeschen K, T Gruner, E Saling: Z Geburtsh u Perinat 188 (1984) 12

(16) Hammacher K, R Brun del Re, R Gaudenz, P De Grandi, R Richter: Gynäkol Rdsch 14 (Suppl 1) (1974) 61

(17) Havercamp D, M Orleans, S Langendoerfer, J McFee, J Murphy, HE Thompson: Am J Obstet Gynecol 134 (1979) 399

(18) Kubli F, D Berg, G Köhnlein, J Hüter, D Bretz: Geburtsh u Frauenheilk 26 (1966) 1537

(19) Lübbers DW: In: Gänshirt H: Der Hirnkreislauf. Thieme, Stuttgart 1972

(20) Mann LI, A Carmichael, S Duchin: Am J Obstet Gynecol 39 (1972) 726

(21) McIntire MS, WH Pearse: Am J Obstet Gynecol 89 (1964) 540

(22) O'Connor MC, FE Hytten, GD Zanelli: Lancet II (1979) 947

(23) Philip AGS: Lancet II (1979) 1189

(24) Rooth G, R McBride, BJ Ivy: Acta Obstet Gynec Scand 52 (1973) 47

(25) Rooth G, O Fall, R Huch, A Huch: Lancet I (1980) 369

(26) Saling E: In: Huntingford PJ, KA Hüter, E Saling: Perinatal Medicine (1st European Congress, Berlin 1968). Thieme, Stuttgart and Academic Press, New York-London 1969

(27) Saling E: Gynaecologia 160 (1965) 133
(28) Saling E: J Reprod Med 1 (1968) 331
(29) Saling E: Bull Soc Roy Belge Gynec Obstet 38 (1968) 289
(30) Saling E: Fortschr Med 88 (1970) 211
(31) Saling E: Modern Trends in Paediatrics 3 (1970) 51
(32) Saling E: In: Huntingford PJ, RW Beard, FE Hytten, JW Scopes (eds.): Perinatal Medicine (2nd Europ Cong Perinat Med, London 1970). Karger, Basel 1971
(33) Saling E: In: Dudenhausen JW, E Saling (eds.): Perinatale Medizin Bd IV. Thieme, Stuttgart 1973
(34) Saling E: Lancet I (1980) 370
(35) Saling E: In: Dudenhausen JW, E Saling (eds.): Periantale Medizin Bd X. Thieme, Stuttgart 1984
(36) Saling E: In: Rooth G, OD Saugstad (eds.): The Roots of Perinatal Medicine. Thieme, Stuttgart 1985
(37) Teramo K: Gynaecologia 167 (1969) 511

BIOCHEMICAL MONITORING OF INTRAPARTUM FETUS

Molly S. Chatterjee, M.D.

Associate Prof., New York Medical College, Chief, Maternal Fetal Medicine, Our Lady of Mercy Medical Center, and Chief Maternal Fetal Medicine, Catholic Medical Center of Brooklyn and Queens, Major Affiliate of New York Hospital - Cornell University.

Electronic Fetal Monitoring is being used worldwide since late 1960's. It was realized that cardiotocography needs to be complemented by biochemical monitoring to identify a fetus in stress from the fetus in distress. At the same time fetal blood sampling of intrapartum fetus for blood gas analysis was introduced by Saling. This fetal capillary blood sampling was practiced only in selected centers throughout the world and never gained popularity for the following reasons:

1) Intermittent serial sampling necessary.
2) Lack of proper training.
3) Lack of availability of blood gas analyser which is able to analyse a microsample (10, 1).
4) Potential risk of bleeding and infection.

It has been noted, since 1978, 16% of the rise in the cesarean rate was attributed to fetal distress. In 1978, only 1.1% of charts listed fetal distress as an accompanying diagnosis. Whereas, in 1984, it increased to 10.4%. This increase may be due to a change in definitions of these complications to include less severe forms. Thus, National Institute of Child Health and Human Development (NICHD) sudy recommends developing additional efforts to define diagnostic classes of fetal distress. There is no doubt that liberal use of fetal scalp sampling can refine the diagnosis of fetal distress as shown by Saling and his co-workers (1987). If only electronic fetal heart rate monitoring is performed, the rate of operative delivery, especially cesarean section is approximately twice as shown by the above workers. Even with combination of cardiotocography and fetal scalp blood sampling the diagnosis of fetal distress during labor remains imprecise. Combination of only these two techniques reported false positive

Dedicated to my father M. M. Ghosh, who encouraged me to pick up the field of perinatal medicine

diagnosis of fetal distress in 71 to 95% of fetuses and detected by 46-61% of distressed fetuses. Therefore, combination of more than one biochemical marker to diagnose fetal distress is necessary to improve the diagnosis of fetal distress.
Electronic heart rate monitoring has a high false positive rate which needs to be evaluated by fetal biochemical monitoring to reduce the risks of operative delivery of the mother. Labor is a stress to the fetus as shown by different workers. There could be changes in the fetal heart rate patterns due to surge of catecholamines in the normal intrapartum fetus. Development of transient respiratory acidosis or more ominous metabolic acidosis in the fetus can only be identified by biochemical monitoring of the fetus. The biochemical fetal parameters that have been and are being studied so far are:

1) Intermittent capillary pH.
2) Continuous tissue pH.
3) Continuous transcutaneous PCO_2.
4) Continuous transcutaneous PO_2.
5) Continuous base excess.
6) Lactate.

It is the purpose of this chapter to introduce the techniques of measurement and details of these fetal biochemical markers and the future of this high technology.
<u>Intermittent Capillary pH</u> - This parameter was first introduced by Saling. Introduction of Corometrics 220 pH meter at bedside has simplified the measurement process. Intermittent sampling, however, has failed to gain popularity inspite of the simplicity of the technique. Lack of adequate education and training may be partly responsible for this unpopularity. A continuous method of biochemical monitoring of the fetus was then sought for.
<u>Continuous Tissue pH</u> - Since late 1970 a glass electrode was introduced to study continuous fetal tissue pH. Due to extreme invasive nature of the electrode and complications associated with it, it was abandoned in a few years. Since early 1980 development of the fiber optic probe has generated renewed interest among researchers in this field. International Biomedics has developed a new monitor called fetascan 1500, which has incorporated the fiberoptic principle to monitor continuous tissue pH in the fetus by a scalp electrode. At the time of this writing,

about 500 cases have been monitored by this improved technology and the future seems to be promising because of its continuous nature and simplicity of the technique. A correlation coefficient of 0.8 has been obtained between tissue pH, capillary pH, and umbilical arterial pH monitored by this method.

Continuous Monitoring of Transcutaneous Carbon Dioxide - Recently fetal transcutaneous carbon dioxide (TcPCO2) measurements have been reported. These investigations have shown very good correlation between TcPCO2 and PCO_2 in samples of capillary blood and umbilical arterial blood. The electrode is applied when the cervical dilatation is at least 3 cm and the membranes are ruptured. Calibration is done with 5% and 10% gas mixture at 44°C. A chemical sensor (Radiometer TCM200) fixed on fetal presenting part by a plastic suction ring by means of negative pressure of 160 mm Hg. has been used to monitor transcutaneous PCO_2. Preliminary results of this electrode function are encouraging. The noninvasive nature of this technique has tremendous appeal. This method has been used in USA, Denmark, and West Germany.

Continuous Base Excess - Simultaneous continuous monitoring of acid base state by TcPCO2 and tissue pH measurements would elucidate the nature of the fetal acisosis during labor. Since base excess is a mathematical manipulation of pH and PCO_2 this parameter has been measured by using Sigaard Anderson nomogram or computerised program. This parameter reflects the ominous type of metabolic acidosis which necessitates expedited delivery.

Continuous Transcutaneous PO2 - Reports of transcutaneous PO_2 monitoring have come mostly from European centers. Electrodes have been developed by some centers which are capable of monitoring fetal ECG and PO_2 (tissue!) simultaneously.

All these technical developments are still in the experimental stage. Further work is necessary to advocate measurement of these biochemical fetal markers to refine the diagnosis of fetal distress. The diagnosis of fetal distress during labor remains imprecise by combination of cardiotocography fetal scalp blood sampling and umbilical cord blood sampling (Saling, 1987).

Lactate - Lactate determinations are mostly restricted to cord blood analysis as of 1987. About 200 1 of fetal blood is necessary for lactate determination, as a result it is impractical to attempt to study this parameter in the fetus. Future development of tchnology is necessary before human fetal lactate estimation can be attempted with minimal amount of fetal capillary blood in the intrapartum period.

It is proposed that future fetal blood monitoring should have 6 channels with continuous monitoring of PO_2, PCO_2, base excess, tissue pH along with cardiotocography, before this high technology can be properly evaluated.

The fiberoptic tissue pH electrode is a major development in the field of intrapartum fetal monitoring. The continuous transcutaneous PCO_2 electrode is very simple to apply by suction fixation. It has been demonstrated by the Danish group that the suction ring does not interfere with the measured value when compared with glue fixation. The latter method was used in West German by Schmidt. The suction fixation is a more popular method of application and is being used at USA in our center at the time of this writing. The continuous recording is easily documented and can be correlated with fetal heart rate patterns.

Metabolic acidosis with lactic acid formation is more ominous than respiratory acidosis. Thus, the base excess, defined as the difference in concentration of strong base between the blood and the same blood titrated with strong acid or base to pH 7.40 and PCO2 40 mm of hg at 37°C is the negative value of the amount of nonvolatile acid, mainly lactic acid. Knowing the PCO2 and the pH of blood, the base excess can be calculated by nomogram or Sigaard-Anderson formula.

There is no doubt that combination of continuous monitoring methods of the fetus during labor are far superior to single estimation or intermittent estimations alone. Thus, attempts are being made to continuously monitor the intrapartum fetus. Currently these monitoring methods are reserved only in research centers in Europe and USA. Further technical developments are necessary before these techniques can be applied for routine clinical use. One possibly could be optimistic and predict such routine clinical use in the near future.

References

(1) Chatterjee M, F Hetzel, H Kaminetzky: Fetal tissue pH - continuous intrapartum monitoring. Int J Gynecol Obstet 22 (1984) 41
(2) Chatterjee M: Proceedings of third Asia-Oceania Congress in Perinatology, Elsevier. Intrapartum Biochemical Monitoring Editor-Maede (in press)
(3) van den Berg P, S Schmidt, J Gesche, E Saling: Fetal distress and the condition of the newborn using cardiotocography and fetal blood analysis during labor. Br J Obstet Gynaecol 94 (1987) 72
(4) Chatterjee M (ed.) Intrapartum Biochemical Monitoring. Walter de Gruyter, Berlin-New York 1988
(5) Nickelsen C, G Sten, T and T Weber: Continuous acid base assessment of the human fetus during labor by tissue pH and transcutaneous carbon dioxide monitoring. Br J Obstet Gynecol 92 (1985) 220

THE RATIONALE FOR BIOCHEMICAL MONITORING OF THE FETUS

MOLLY E. TOWELL

Department of Obstetrics and Gynecology, McMaster University
Hamilton, Ontario, Canada

Although our understanding of the pathophysiology of birth asphyxia has increased considerably over the last twenty-five years, the effects of asphyxia on brain development remain controversial. In this paper I will deal with the definition and incidence of birth asphyxia, the etiology of intrapartum asphyxia and the outcome measures which have been used in randomized controlled trials of fetal intensive care. In addition, I will discuss the relationship of birth asphyxia to the subsequent development of hypoxic-ischaemic encephalopathy and cerebral palsy.

1. The Definition and Incidence of Birth Asphyxia

The definition of asphyxia as given in Webster's New World Dictionary is "loss of consciousness as a result of too little oxygen and too much carbon dioxide in the blood." Thus, the dictionary gives both a biochemical and a biophysical definition. The biochemical definition can be precisely determined in terms of pH, PCO_2 and PO_2 and usually takes the form of a combined respiratory and metabolic acidosis. However, a biophysical definition, i.e., the Apgar scoring system, has been widely used for many years exclusive of any biochemical definition.

The true incidence of birth asphyxia is difficult to determine from the literature. Only those papers in which consecutive deliveries were reported are considered here so that bias from inclusion or exclusion of specific data is avoided. Table 1 shows the results of studies which satisfy these criteria and in which a biochemical definition for birth asphyxia was used, based on the pH of umbilical cord blood at birth.

It can be seen from Table 1 that the incidence of birth asphyxia depends on the precise pH chosen to define acidosis. If the definition used is that of pH < 7.1, the incidence varies from 2.3% to 8.6%, whereas, if the definition is widened to pH < 7.2, the incidence varies from 4.8% to 21.6%. There seems to have been consistent improvement in the incidence of low pH at birth over the years between 1972 and 1987. This is particularly evident in the figures obtained from Dr. Saling's unit (2,5). Indeed, the recent figures emerging from their unit show that less than 5% of babies are now born with a UA pH of less than 7.2.

Table I Incidence of Birth Asphyxia in Consecutive Deliveries Based on Umbilical Cord Blood pH

Source	n	UA/UV	Mean ± SD	Low pH
Kubli 1972(1)	3317	UA	7.26(median)	<7.2 -21.1% <7.1 - 4.4%
Boenisch & Saling 1974(2)	5724	UA	-	<7.2 -10.6% <7.1 - 2.3%
Sykes et al 1982(3)	899	UA	7.20 ± .08	<7.1 - 8.6%
MacDonald et al 1985(4)	1075	UV	7.30 ± .07	<7.1 - 1.5%
van den Berg et al 1987(5)	2669	UA	7.30 ± .07	<7.2 - 4.8%

UA=umbilical artery UV=umbilical vein

An exception is the data of Sykes et al (3) which shows the highest incidence of acidosis (pH < 7.1) of all the studies. However, it is possible that methodological errors may account for their low pH values since pH was not always measured immediately after collection of blood samples.

It is difficult to compare the data from MacDonald et al (4) with the remainder of the data in Table 1 since the vessel chosen for blood sampling was the umbilical vein. Umbilical venous blood will not provide a satisfactory measure of acidosis in the fetus particularly under conditions of umbilical cord compression (see later) and the low incidence of acidosis reported by this group in over 1000 consecutive deliveries may reflect this problem.

It can be concluded that there are a number of problems in the biochemical definition of birth asphyxia. Firstly, if pH is to be used as the criteria, there is no agreement on the absolute value of pH which should be considered as abnormal. Should we use a pH value of 7.2 or 7.1 and should we use other parameters in addition such as PO_2, O_2 saturation, PCO_2 or lactate values? Secondly, if umbilical cord blood is used in the biochemical determination, the duration of asphyxia is not known and there is no clear indication of whether the acidosis is chronic and long-standing or has developed acutely over the last few minutes of labour and delivery. The long-term prognosis of these two situations may be entirely different, and continuous biochemical monitoring may be the only way to monitor the duration of an asphyxial episode.

In many centres a biophysical score, usually the Apgar score or a modification of Apgar score, is the only criterion used for a diagnosis of birth asphyxia. The data which has been obtained from consecutive deliveries has been examined (Table 2), and there are wide variations in the definition and incidence using a low Apgar score, similar to those found using pH to define asphyxia.

Table 2 Incidence of Birth Asphyxia Defined by Apgar Score

Source	n	Apgar	%
Drage et al 1964(6)	10,020	<7 at 5 min	4.0%
Boenisch & Saling 1974(1)	5,724	<7 at 1.5 min	6.7%
Sykes et al 1982(2)	895	<4 at 1 min	3.8%
Macdonald et al 1985(4)	13,084	<4 at 1 or 5 min	1.0%
van den Berg et al 1987(5)	2,669	<7 at 1.5 min	1.05%

The definition of birth asphyxia by Apgar score is complicated by the presence of both false positives and false negatives (7,8). False positives (low Apgar and normal pH) can be seen with prematurity, analgesia, anaesthesia, trauma at delivery and congenital malformations. False negatives (normal Apgar and low pH) can be seen with short term asphyxia, chronic asphyxia in which fetal adaptation has occurred, and maternal metabolic acidosis.

A combined scoring system using both low Apgar score and low pH has been advocated by some authors (2, 5) and the results of three studies in which this combined approach to scoring at birth has been used is shown in Table 3; again, only those papers in which consecutive deliveries were studied are presented here. This type of approach in which not only the biochemical definition of asphyxia is used but also the effect on the fetus and newborn is taken into consideration, seems to be the most logical one in that it considers the functional effects of the biochemical abnormality.

Table 3 Incidence of Birth Asphyxia Defined as Low pH and Low Apgar in Consecutive Deliveries

	Low UA pH	Low Apgar	Low pH + Low Apgar
Boenisch & Saling 1974(2)	<7.2 10.6%	<7 at 1.5 min 6.7%	3.2%
Sykes et al 1982(3)	<7.1 8.5%	<7 at 1 min 10.8%	2.2%
van den Berg 1987(5)	<7.2 4.8%	<7 at 1.5 min 1.5%	0.7%

2. Etiology of Intrapartum Birth Asphyxia

The underlying cause of birth asphyxia is impaired placental gas exchange and the common pathological events leading to this situation during the intrapartum course are listed in Table 4.

Not included in this list are problems which precede the intrapartum course such as acute or chronic maternal hypertension, maternal or fetal cardiac failure, intrauterine growth failure and placental insufficiency. However, impairment of placental exchange before the onset of labour will considerably increase the intrapartum risk of asphyxia.

Table 4 Intrapartum Causes of Birth Asphyxia

1. Reduction of Uterine Blood Flow
   e.g. increased uterine activity
   maternal hypotension

2. Reduction of Umbilical Blood Flow
   e.g. umbilical cord compression

3. Combined Reduction of Maternal-Fetal Blood Flow
   e.g. abruptio placenta
   second stage (increased uterine activity
   ± cord compression)

There is usually a decline in pH during the course of labour and particularly during the second stage. Kubli (1) showed that there was a shift in median pH from 7.31 in early first stage to slightly lower values in late first stage. Median values for the second stage were 7.25 with a wide scattering of values below 7.1. Our own data, obtained from a small group of healthy women (n=28) in normal labour who were followed throughout first and second stages with multiple fetal blood samples, showed a similar decline in pH in the second stage of labour (Figure 1).

Fetal pH fell from a mean of 7.30 in scalp blood samples during labour to 7.24 in umbilical cord blood at birth. It should be noted that pH was well maintained throughout the first stage and even early second stage, only falling when the second stage had been in progress for more than thirty minutes. Note that maternal pH also fell during the second stage due to the development of a mild metabolic acidosis without any change in PCO_2, presumably due to lactic acidosis from the physical activity involved in bearing down efforts. In contrast, the acidosis which developed in the fetus was due to a combination of respiratory and metabolic acidosis (Figure 1).

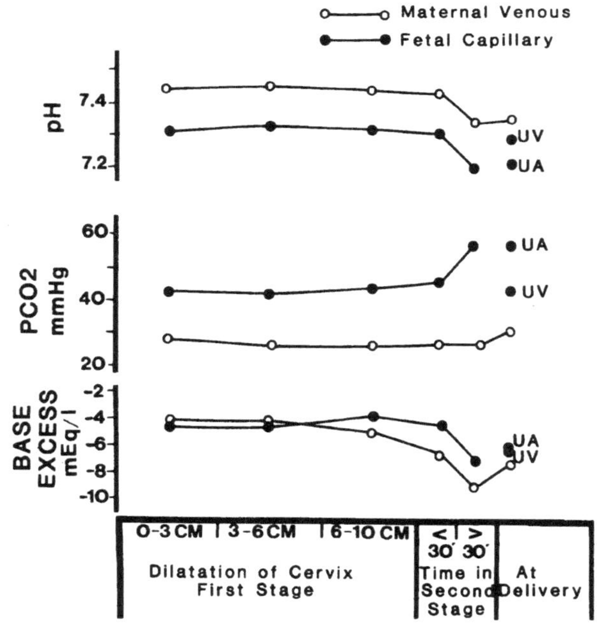

Figure 1 Mean values for pH, PCO_2 and base excess in maternal venous and fetal capillary (scalp) blood during normal labour and delivery in a group of healthy women (n=28). UA = umbilical artery; UV = umbilical vein.

Umbilical cord entanglement which was present in about 34% of 749 patients monitored in labour in our own data, is probably the commonest cause of fetal acidosis. pH values in umbilical arterial blood were significantly lower when cord entanglement was present (Table 5), although there was no difference in umbilical venous blood pH.

The explanation for maintenance of umbilical venous blood pH in the presence of umbilical cord compression is that maternal blood flow through the placenta remains uninterrupted while reduced blood flow through the umbilical circulation can satisfactorily maintain exchange with the mother at least in the early phases of cord compression. As a consequence of this, there is a significantly wider difference in pH between umbilical arterial and venous blood when cord complications are present (Table 5).

Table 5 Umbilical Arterial (UA) and Umbilical Venous (UV) Blood pH (mean ± SD) at Birth in the Presence or Absence of Cord Entanglement

	Cord Entanglement		
	Absent n=473	Present n=246	
UA pH	7.29 ± .074	7.26 ± 0.098	p<0.005
UV pH	7.35 ± .068	7.35 ± 0.077	n.s.
UV-UA pH	0.06 ± .034	0.08 ± .054	p<0.001

Cord compression has also been studied in fetal lambs (9). Figure 2 shows results from experiments in fetal lambs at 127 to 142 days gestation in which the umbilical cord was mildly compressed for a period of thirty minutes. The anticipated changes in pH, PO_2, PCO_2 and lactate can be seen from Figure 2 although the degree of compression was such that pH only fell from 7.36 to 7.26 during the thirty minute period. Changes in fetal brain electrocortical (ECoG) activity, although not significantly different, showed a trend towards increased high voltage activity during cord compression which promptly reverted to a normal percentage of time spent in high voltage and low voltage activity in the post-compression period. This suggests that even mild degrees of asphyxia may be accompanied by changes in functional activity of brain cells.

In one experiment in a fetal lamb, the umbilical cord was severely compressed for a period of twelve minutes. Figure 3 shows portions of the electrocortical (ECoG) activity from the fetal brain before, during and after compression. It can be seen that ECoG activity disappeared completely at 2-3 minutes after the start of cord compression i.e., at a time when pH had only fallen from 7.39 to 7.30. The most significant change during this period was a dramatic fall in PO_2 from 25.6 to 5.5 mm Hg within two minutes of compression.

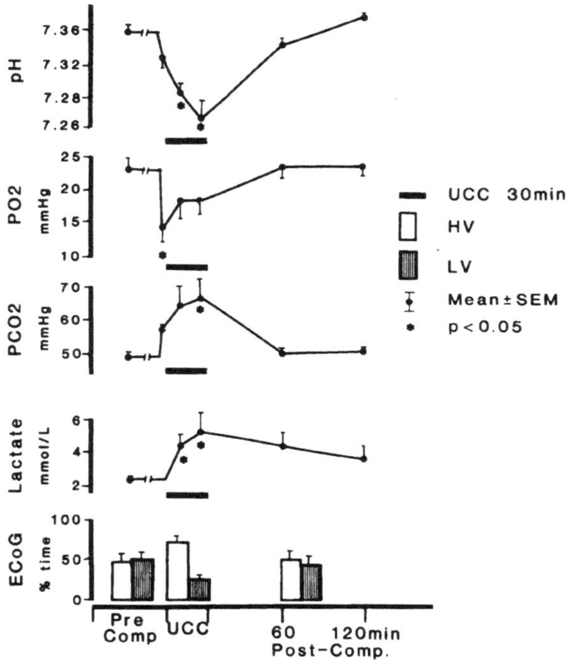

Figure 2 Effects of mild umbilical cord compression on fetal acid-base state and electrocortical (ECoG) activity in three fetal lambs at 127-142 days gestation. All experiments performed at >7 days after surgical preparation.

There was also a very large increase in lactate which only slowly resolved following compression. Lactate values remained elevated for at least three hours after the cord was released, presumably due to the slow washout of lactate from tissues once peripheral circulation was re-established during recovery from asphyxia. Similarly ECoG activity showed a slow return to its normal cyclical pattern of high voltage and low voltage activity. It is anticipated that experiments of this type will help to show how the biochemical defect in asphyxia impinges on tissue function and could provide valuable insight into the normal recovery patterns of cellular function.

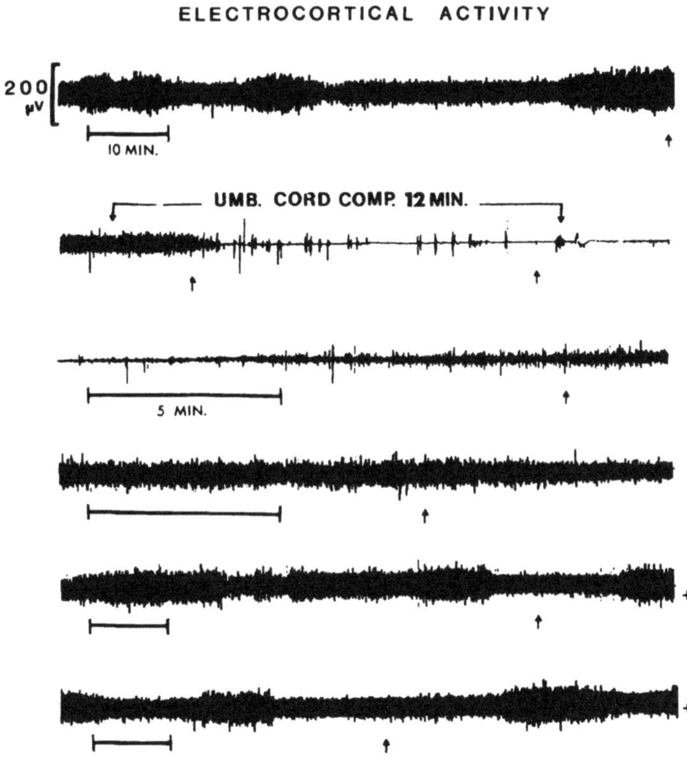

FETAL ARTERIAL BLOOD

	pH	PCO2 mmHg	PO2 mmHg	Lactate mmol/L
PRE	7.39	48.5	25.6	2.6
U.C.C.				
2'	7.30	64.5	5.5	3.8
11'	6.84	139.0	5.0	12.5
POST				
+15'	7.04	72.6	21.5	12.1
+60'	7.26	46.7	23.5	10.4
+120'	7.34	47.6	23.1	7.9
+180'	7.38	42.6	22.0	6.8

Figure 3 Electrocortical activity, pH, PCO_2, PO_2 and lactate measurements in a fetal lamb at 133 days gestation before, during and after a 12 minute period of umbilical cord compression (U.C.C.). Arrows indicate arterial blood samples.

3. Outcome Measures in Birth Asphyxia

The effects of birth asphyxia are listed in Table 6 as modified from Fomufod et al (10) and deSa (11). Although the effects of asphyxia on the metabolism and the central nervous system are the most obvious at birth, there may be multi-organ dysfunction with widespread effects on bone marrow, kidneys, lungs, gastrointestinal tract and cardiovascular system in as many as 76% of infants affected (10). Widespread ischaemic damage may culminate in neonatal death or death in early infancy.

Table 6 — Effects of Intrapartum Asphyxia on the Fetus and the Newborn Infant

Metabolic
- metabolic acidosis, hypoglycemia, hypocalcemia, hyponatremia

CNS
- hypoxic-ischaemic encephalopathy
- neonatal seizures
- brain swelling
- long term neurological handicaps

Haematologic
- thrombocytopenia, DIC

Renal Damage

Pulmonary
- hyaline membrane disease
- persistent fetal circulation

Gastrointestinal
- necrotizing enterocolitis
- liver dysfunction

Cardiovascular
- bradycardia, hyper/hypotension
- myocardial necrosis

Perinatal Death

Modified from Fomufod et al (10); deSa (11)

Much of the effort in obstetrical perinatal care over the past two decades has been directed towards development of sophisticated monitoring technics for fetal intensive care during labour. To date, the results of most randomized controlled trials using continuous fetal heart rate monitoring as a method of preventing perinatal asphyxia have been disappointing. Table

7 lists those studies which conform to the stringent criteria of truly randomized controlled trials. As can be seen, there have been no significant differences in any of the trials to date in either perinatal mortality or Apgar score.

Table 7 Randomized Controlled Trials of Continuous Fetal Heart Rate Monitoring

Source	Year	n	Perinatal Mortality	Apgar Score	Umbilical Arterial Blood pH	Neurol-ogical Outcome
Haverkamp et al(12)	1976	483	n.s	n.s	n.s	n.s
Haverkamp et al(13)	1978	695	n.s	n.s	n.s	n.s
Renou et al(14)	1976	344	n.s	n.s	$p<0.05^1$	$p<0.001$
Kelso et al(15)	1978	504	n.s	n.s	"no diff."	n.s
MacDonald et al(4)	1985	12,964	n.s	n.s	n.s[2]	$p=0.025$

n.s = not significant [1] n = 86 [2] n = 1000; umbilical venous blood

pH has only been shown to be significantly different in one study in which pH was lower in unmonitored patients; however, the number of patients involved was small. It is unfortunate that in the Dublin randomized controlled trial (4) involving the largest number of patients, only 1000 of their patients were evaluated with umbilical cord blood pH and the vessel chosen was the umbilical vein and not the umbilical artery. Thus, no conclusions can be drawn from their data regarding the effect of monitoring on the biochemical outcome for the fetus.

In contrast, neurologic outcome has been shown to be significantly different in at least two trials (4, 14) with a higher incidence of jitteriness and early neonatal seizures in unmonitored patients. It should be noted that, in the Dublin randomized controlled trial (4), biochemical assessment of the fetus was permitted in both arms of the study. Thus, the difference in neurologic outcome was attributed to the application of continuous fetal heart rate monitoring and not to the use of fetal blood sampling.

The data from randomized controlled trials suggests that perinatal mortality and Apgar score will not be useful measures of outcome in any future trial of fetal intensive care. The current low level of perinatal mortality and its multiple etiology make it a poor choice as an outcome measure for birth asphyxia. Similarly, Apgar score alone, because of high false negative and false positive rates in relation to fetal acidosis, is not a good measure for the presence or absence of birth asphyxia. The presence of fetal acidosis unrelated to maternal acidosis is diagnostic of impaired placental exchange and should be included in a definition of birth asphyxia. However, the absence of fetal acidosis does not exclude the possibility that episodes of asphyxia, from which the fetus has since recovered, may have preceded labour and delivery. Finally, neurologic outcome can be regarded as an important outcome measure to which we should pay close attention in the future.

Although Apgar score may not be a good measure of birth asphyxia, it is the only one that has been used for many years and a large volume of data available from the National Collaborative Perinatal Project (1955-1966) has been based on this outcome measure. Apgar scores were recorded in approximately 49,000 infants at 1 and 5 minutes and the presence or absence of cerebral palsy was known in 37,000 children who were available for follow up at 7 years of age. This data was subsequently analyzed by Nelson and Ellenberg (16) and the development of cerebral palsy compared with Apgar score at birth. The mortality rate was very high for infants <2500 gm at the time this data was collected. Furthermore, the etiology of cerebral palsy in low birth weight infants is known to be correlated with postnatal as well as prenatal factors. For these reasons, I have only considered their data from term infants of >2500 gm. Infants with very low Apgar scores of 0-3 showed an increasing mortality during the first year of life and an increasing morbidity (cerebral palsy) related to the latest time interval after birth at which an Apgar score of 0-3 was recorded (Table 8). It should be noted, however, that of the 120 children known to have cerebral palsy at 7 years of age which was not acquired postnatally, 55% had Apgar scores of 7-10 at 1 minute and 73% had scores of 7-10 at 5 minutes. Since the majority of infants will have normal Apgar scores at birth, the largest single group of children with cerebral palsy can be expected to come from this group, while a minority will come from groups with low Apgar scores.

It is clear from this data that a severely depressed infant at birth, particularly one that remains depressed and does not respond to resuscitation, has an increased risk of cerebral palsy related to the time interval over which it remains depressed after birth. However, many infants show no signs of birth asphyxia as judged by the Apgar score and it is therefore unlikely that their subsequent developmental problems can be attributed to intrapartum asphyxia. Indeed, it is more likely that, in this group, the cause of cerebral palsy antedates the intrapartum period and may or may not be related to asphyxia. The probability that factors preceding labour and delivery are very important in subsequent development of cerebral palsy has been pointed out by a multivariate analysis of the data from the National Collaborative Perinatal Project (17). This analysis showed that maternal mental retardation, birth weight below 2001 grams and fetal malformation were among the leading predictors of cerebral palsy.

Table 8 Apgar Scores and Outcome by Latest Very Low Apgar Score (0-3) (> 2500 gm)

Apgar 0-3 (time-mins)	Liveborn	Death in First Yr (%)	Known to 7 Yrs.	With Cerebral Palsy (%)
1	1729	3.1	1330	0.7
5	286	7.7	217	0.9
10	66	18.2	43	4.7
15	23	47.8	11	9.1
20	39	59.0	14	57.1

From Nelson & Ellenberg, 1981 (16)

Breech presentation was also a predictor although breech delivery was not. Forty of the 189 survivors with cerebral palsy had evidence of birth asphyxia as judged by low Apgar score at birth. However, 23/40 or 57.5% had other factors present which were predetermined before the onset of labour such as birth weight below 2001 grams, congenital malformation etc. This data supports the idea that many fetuses are already predestined to develop cerebral palsy even before the onset of labour and that intrapartum asphyxia is responsible for a relatively small percentage of infants who eventually show neurologic developmental problems.

In 1982, Dennis and Chalmers (18) proposed that very early neonatal seizure rate could be used as a strong indicator of the quality of care based on their analysis of babies who developed seizures in the first forty-eight hours of life. They suggested that morbidity indices should be based on neonatal clinical signs which were unambiguous and strongly predictive of later morbidity such as cerebral palsy. Thus they proposed that the frequency of neonatal seizures in the first forty-eight hours of life should be considered as an index which met these criteria with respect to full term babies. The analysis of data from randomized controlled trials also suggested that, although the seizure rate did not achieve statistical significance in most of the studies, there was a trend towards a higher seizure rate in the unmonitored group. Thus, the Dublin randomized controlled trial was designed to use neonatal seizures as an outcome measure. Table 9 reproduced from that study (4) shows that there were twice as many infants with early neonatal seizures in the control (auscultated) group as in the electronic fetal monitoring group ($p < 0.025$) and the neonatal death rate following development of seizures was also twice as high ($p < 0.05$).

Table 9 Dublin RCT of Intrapartum Electronic Fetal Monitoring (EFM)

Sequelae of Neonatal Seizures	EFM	Auscultation	Significance
Neonatal death	3	6	$p < 0.05$
Survival	9	21	
Total no. of seizures	12	27	$p < 0.025$
Relative Risk (95% confid.)	.45	1.0	

From MacDonald et al. (4)

Hypoxic-ischaemic encephalopathy (HIE) is the term used to identify the cerebral problems in the full term infant following intrapartum or neonatal asphyxia. The pathological lesions are located in the peripheral and dorsal areas of the cerebral cortex and involve necrosis of the gyri at the depths of the sulci and neuronal nuclei of the basal ganglia and brain stem (19). The clinical features of HIE have been classified by Sarnat and Sarnat (20) into three stages: stage I - hyperalert: stage II - lethargic and hypotonic; stage III - stuporous and flaccid. In a careful follow up of survivors to 3.5 years of age, Robertson and Finer (21) used a similar classification into mild, moderate and severe HIE. They showed that none of the mild HIE cases died and none were handicapped at follow up (Table 10). However, with moderate and severe HIE, mortality and morbidity rates progressively increased with severity of the disorder and all survivors in the severe HIE group were handicapped.

Table 10 Outcome to 3.5 Yrs after Hypoxic-Ischaemic Encephalopathy in 226 Term Infants

HIE	n	(Lost to Follow-up)	Deaths In Hosp.	Deaths Later	Follow-up at 3.5 Yrs Not Hand.	Follow-up at 3.5 Yrs Handicapped
Mild	79	(10)	-	-	69	-
Moderate	119	(16)	3	3*	75	22
Severe	28	(0)	14	7	-	7

* 1 death from MVA

From Robertson & Finer (21)

The type of handicap described by Robertson and Finer (21) ranged from cognitive delay (58%), to cerebral palsy (53%), convulsive disorders (34%), visual loss (29%) and deafness

(11%). Thus the development of moderate or severe HIE within the first few days of life is a strong indicator of perinatal asphyxia and of subsequent morbidity.

Finally, the follow up study by Low et al (22) is the only one to date which relates careful intrapartum monitoring including acid base measurements with subsequent follow up of the child and neurologic assessment. They determined the development of intrapartum asphyxia by a measure of umbilical arterial blood buffer base and they classified their deficits at one year follow up as major or minor, motor and/or cognitive problems and showed an increasing incidence of deficits as buffer base values declined from 34 mmol/l to <22 mmol/l (Figure 4).

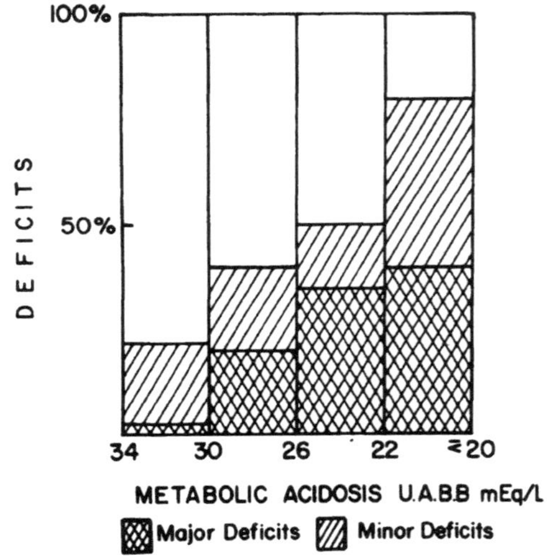

Figure 4 The incidence of major or minor, motor and/or cognitive deficits increased from 20% to 80% as the umbilical artery buffer base decreased from 30-34 to <22 mEq/l. (Reproduced with permission granted by C.V. Mosby Co. From Low, J.A. et al 1984 Am. J. Obstet. Gynecol. 148, 533-539.)

Summary

1. Rates for perinatal mortality and low Apgar scores have not been affected by fetal intensive care (electronic monitoring ± fetal blood sampling) in any randomized controlled trial to date.

2. Acidosis at birth may be susceptible to improvement by fetal intensive care but has not been tested adequately in more than a few women.
3. Birth asphyxia which is followed by evidence of cerebral dysfunction within the first 48 hours of life can be significantly altered by current technics of fetal intensive care.
4. The evidence suggests that cognitive disorders and cerebral palsy occur as long term sequelae of hypoxic-ischaemic encephalopathy in a small percentage of survivors. However, factors which predate the onset of labour are more likely to be responsible for cerebral palsy than factors associated with labour.
5. Future developments might include the following:
(i) To establish that umbilical arterial pH and/or lactate and/or Apgar score is predictive for neonatal outcome such as hypoxic-ischaemic encephalopathy or other markers of asphyxia.
(ii) To determine whether umbilical arterial pH and/or lactate is significantly different when continuous biochemical monitoring is used versus traditional intermittent fetal blood sampling, i.e. does continuous monitoring prevent acidosis?

In the present state of development of continuous biochemical monitoring technics in labour it seems unlikely that, at the present time, we could answer the larger question of whether such monitoring can prevent the neurological complications of hypoxic-ischaemic encephalopathy and the subsequent developmental problems including cerebral palsy.

Finally, we must not forget that labour and delivery represents a relatively small time period in relation to the total duration of pregnancy with a ratio of approximately 1:355. Thus, it is not surprising that many of the problems of neurologic development are difficult to trace back to a particular stage in pregnancy. Careful monitoring of labour and delivery may help to counteract the tendency to blame this period of pregnancy for all subsequent developmental problems of the child.

References

(1) Kubli F: Respiratory gas exchange and blood flow in the placenta. In: Longo LD and H Bartels (eds.): DHEW Publications no. NIH 73-361 (1972) pp 487
(2) Boenisch H, E Saling: J Perinat Med 2 (1974) 122
(3) Sykes GS, P Johnson, F Ashworth, PM Molloy, W Gu, GM Stirrat, AC Turnbull: Lancet 1 (1982) 494
(4) MacDonald D, A Grant, M Sheridan-Pereira, P Boylan, I Chalmers: Am J Obstet Gynecol 152 (1985) 524
(5) van den Berg P, S Schmidt, J Gesche, E Saling: Brit J Obstet & Gynaecol 94 (1987) 72

(6) Drage JS, C Kennedy, DK Schwarz: Obstet Gynecol 24 (1964) 222
(7) Bowe ET, RW Beard, M Firston, PJ Poppers, K Adamsons, LS James: Amer J Obstet Gynecol 107 (1970) 279
(8) Lissauer TJ, PJ Steer: Brit J Obstet Gynaecol 93 (1986) 1060
(9) Dinh T, ME Towell: Unpublished Data (1987)
(10) Fomufod AK, F Rahbar, PL White, AL Holloway, WR Rampersaud, LA Henry: J Nat Med Assoc 71 (1979) 939
(11) deSa DJ: Arch Dis Child 54 (1979) 918
(12) Haverkamp AD, HE Thompson, JG McFee, C Cetrulo: Amer J Obstet Gynecol 125 (1976) 310
(13) Haverkamp AD, M Orleans, S Langendoerfer, J McFee, J Murphy, HE Thompson: Amer J Obstet Gynecol 134 (1979) 399
(14) Renou P, A Chang, I Anderson, C Wood: Amer J Obstet Gynecol 126 (1976) 470
(15) Kelso IM, RJ Parsons, GF Lawrence, SS Arora, DK Edmonds, ID Cooke: Amer J Obstet Gynecol 131 (1978) 526
(16) Nelson KB, JH Ellenberg: Pediatrics 68 (1981) 36
(17) Nelson KB, JH Ellenberg: N Engl J Med 31 (1986) 81
(18) Dennis J, I Chalmers: Brit J Obstet Gynaecol 89 (1982) 418
(19) Brann AW: Ped Clin M America 33 (1986) 451
(20) Sarnat HB, MS Sarnat: Arch Neurol 33 (1976) 696
(21) Robertson C, M Finer: Dev Med & Child Neurol 27 (1985) 473
(22) Low JA, RS Galbraith, DW Muir, HL Killen, EA Pater, EJ Karchmar: Obstet Gynecol 148 (1984) 533

CONTINUOUS INTRAPARTUM FETAL SCALP TISSUE pH AND ECG MONITORING BY A FIBEROPTIC PROBE

Howard M. Hochberg, M.D.
Paul V. Roby, M.D.
Hattie M. Snell, R.N.
W. Dean Smith, B.S.
International Biomedics, Inc., Bothell, Washington 98021

Molly S. Chatterjee, M.D.
Our Lady of Mercy Medical Center, Bronx, N.Y. 10466

Introduction

Labor and delivery can rapidly change from a normal to a potentially high risk situation. Accordingly, careful monitoring of mother and fetus has become the standard of care. Continuous electronic "fetal" monitoring (EFM) of fetal heart rates and uterine contractions is used almost universally in the United States. EFM information is sensitive to the possibility of dangerous deficits in fetal oxygen supply. However EFM data yields about 50 to 60% false positive "diagnoses" of significant fetal hypoxia (1) and may not detect up to 15-20% of true hypoxia. The most specific index of prolonged and potentially dangerous insufficient oxygen delivery is fetal blood pH (BpH); measured from drops of blood carefully collected from a small incision on the fetal scalp. The combination of BpH and EFM data reduces the incidence of false positives, while also improving detection of true problems. These combined data can be used to substantially reduce the Cesarean section rate for fetal distress (1-4). It is estimated that BpH information may be clinically important in up to 25% of patients (3,5).

However, BpH data is not commonly available because of the skills, time, inconvenience and laboratory facilities needed to obtain reliable measurements. Further one BpH measure is insufficient to determine the trend of fetal pH (5). Finally, the tools and methods are primitive and there is some fetal risk (2). For all these reasons, and despite its potential value, BpH has not become the standard of practice in the United States.

The information inherent in the BpH measurement could be made widely available if there were a convenient safe probe to continuously monitor intrapartum fetal pH. This paper describes an investigational fetal pH probe designed to be safe and convenient. *At this time, the goal of the device is to provide reliable fetal pH status and trend data for use as an adjunct to EFM and BpH data for clinical care.*

Historical Perspective

The first fetal pH probe to undergo widespread clinical trials was the Stamm tissue pH (tpH) probe, designed for monitoring the pH of the subcutaneous fluid in the fetal scalp (6,7). Several studies demonstrated the validity of the basic concept of Stamm: human fetal acid-base balance can be monitored and evaluated by continuous monitoring of the scalp tpH (8-12). Clinical utility included a reduction in operative intervention for deliveries (9). However the Stamm device required sterile assembly and charging with sterile reference electrolyte a scalp incision for probe insertion and mastery of a difficult technique for apply and fixing the probe to the fetal scalp. The system was found to be impractical and the technique unreliable for routine clinical use.

In order to help to make these potentially valuable fetal tpH data generally available the authors and clinician investigators are evaluating a system and tpH probe designed to be convenient, safe, and reliable for continuous monitoring of fetal pH status. Fiberoptic, electro-optic, microprocessor and analytic chemistry technologies were integrated to produce a feasibility system designed for evaluation of continuous clinical monitoring of the fetal pH status during labor: The OBpH™ 1000 System. Using the experience gained in monitoring over 300 patients between late 1983 through mid 1985, a total system designed to be convenient and simple for routine use by the clinician was designed and built. The latter system, the OBpH 1500, is in evaluation at this time. This paper describes the OBpH 1500 system and outlines clinical results from the earlier OBpH 1000 system, which used the same tpH probe.

Because this is an unreleased FDA Class III Investigational Devise in evaluation for regulatory purposes, International Biomedics can make no claims regarding safety, effectiveness or utility of the system. Further, it should be understood the device is designed as an adjunct to EFM and fetal scalp blood sampling, not as a total replacement for either measurement. (1987)

System Description

The OBpH 1500 System includes a fetal scalp pH ECG probe, an applicator tool, an electro-optic Interface module, an off-line Calibration chamber, and a fetal monitor for data display (Figures 1,2). The probe is a 22 gauge spiral ECG electrode which includes a fiberoptic-based pH sensor (Fig. 3,4). The probe is applied to the fetal scalp with the same general technique used for spiral ECG electrodes. When properly placed within the scalp, the pH sensor is within the subcutaneous fluid and the probe detects both subcutaneous fluid (tissue) pH and fetal ECG.

The probe is supplied in a sterile pack, with the tpH sensor within pH 7.00 buffer. After insertion of the probe pack and connector into the Interface, and insertion of the Interface into the Calibrator, the probe is automatically warmed, stabilized, stored and calibrated within the sterile pack. PH 7.36 Calibration is begun by depressing a sealed plunger through the cover of the sterile probe pack. The Calibrator checks for problems, confirms the reliability of the calibration, and the probe is ready for use within about 15 minutes. The calibrated probe can be used with confidence for up to 8 hours.

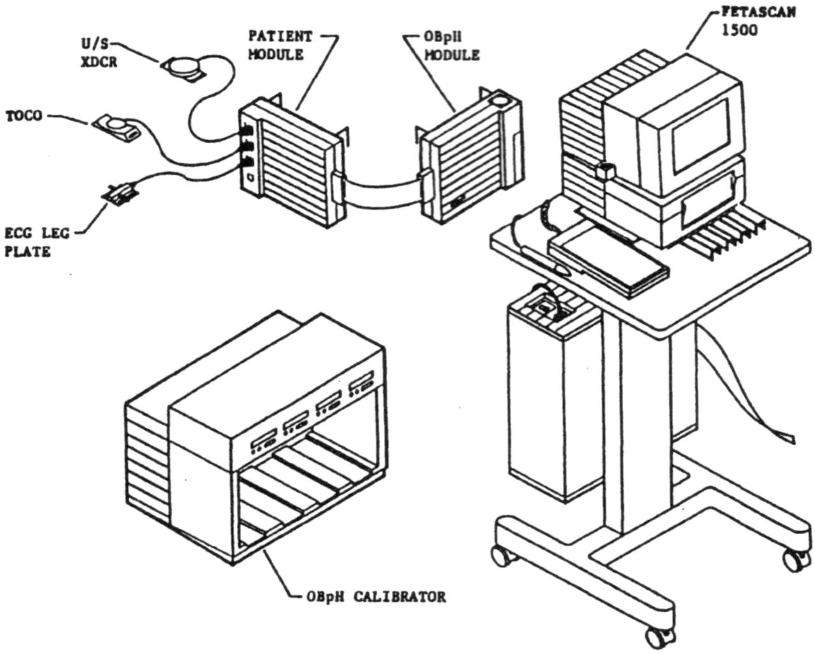

Figure 1 **The OBpH 1500 System**

This illustrates the bedside monitoring configuration of the system. The OBpH Module (Interface), an electro-optic and memory module which can contain the OBpH probe set. The OBpH Interface mates with the Patient Module of the FetaScan 1500. This assembly can be placed at the bedside, as the Patient Module accepts the ECG leg plate cable and uterine contraction transducers and the OBpH Interface can include a calibrated probe ready for use.

The OBpH Interface acquires and retains the probe calibration data, allowing the patient to be disconnected from the monitor for transport by disconnecting the Interface from the Patient Module.

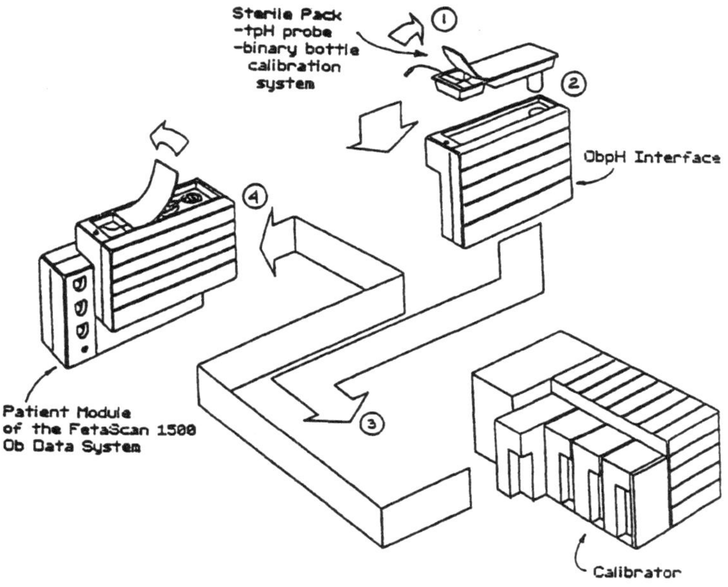

Instructions

(1) Open connector chamber of sterile pack. Insert connector into tpH Interface.

(2) Insert sterile pack into tpH Interface.

(3) Insert tpH interface into Calibrator. Allow for stabilization, calibrate ten minutes before needed.

(4) When calibrated, remove Interface from calibrator, connect Interface to patient module. Probe is ready to use.

Figure 2 **Preparation of the Model 1500 OBpH System**

The OBpH 1500 Interface mates with either the calibrator or the monitor. It acquires and retains the probe calibration data, allowing the patient to be disconnected from and reconnected to any appropriate FetaScan 1500 monitor by disconnecting and reconnecting the interface, without disconnecting the probe.

The OBpH probe is in a sterile sealed package and it can be fully calibrated in this package without impairing sterility. Once calibrated, it can be placed at the bedside ready for use. The semiautomatic Calibrator holds 4 probe-interface packages ready for final calibration and use.

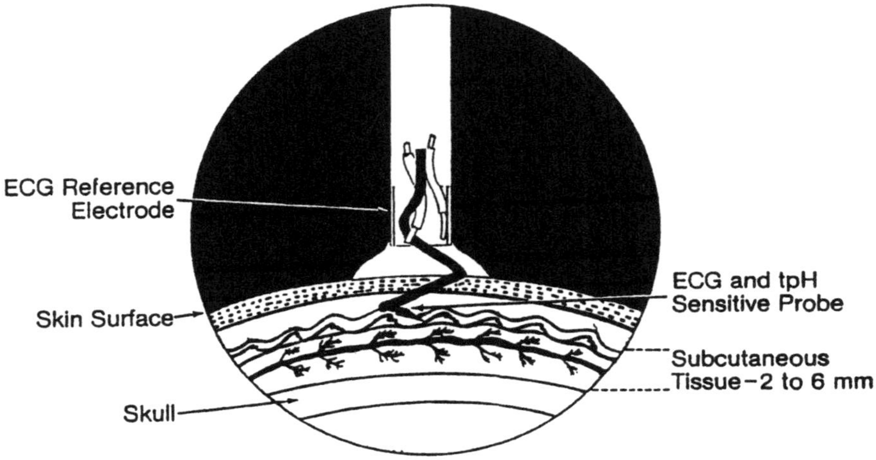

Figure 3

Drawing of the tpH probe in situ in the fetal scalp, with the applicator tool attached. The spiral forms one pole of the ECG electrode and the hub is the other. The tpH sensor window is just below the skin surface, facing into the subcutaneous tissue in order to measure the pH of the interstitial fluid.

Fiberoptic pH Probe Design

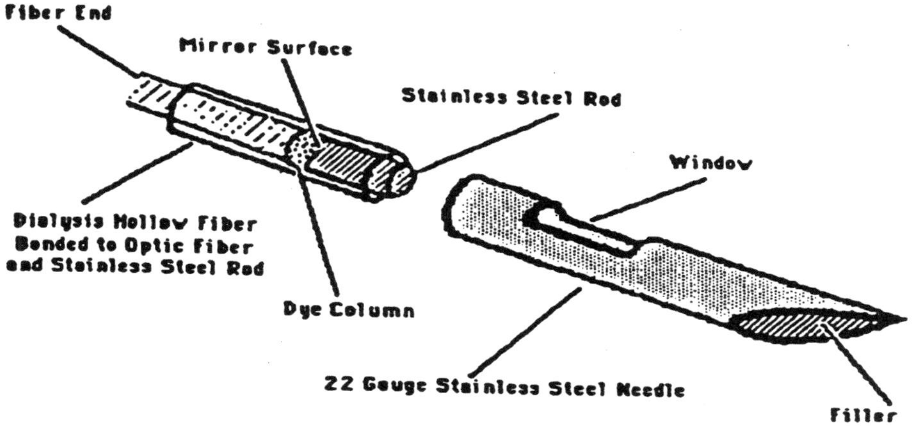

Figure 4 **Principle of Operation of the Fiberoptic pH Probe**

The above assembly is inserted into the solution to be measured. Protons (H+) diffuse freely through the dialysis hollow fiber into the dye column. The column contains a reversible pH-sensitive non-toxic dye covalently bound to a gel matrix (to prevent escape of dye). A fiberoptic fiber guides light to the dye, and directs reflected light to the instrument. There the green reflectance, the red reflectance, and the current with no light (dark current) are measured. The absorbance of green light by the dye is proportional to the pH in the range of interest, while red absorbance is not affected by pH. The red relectance is used as a reference signal.

The Interface module, with probe still attached, is then moved to the bedside. The pack is opened and the probe applied to the fetal scalp. The interface module is then attached to the FetaScan monitor, which automatically acquires and merges the tpH with the monitoring data on its strip chart and the video display, and continuously checks the validity of the optical data in order to flag problems (Fig. 5).

ILLUSTRATIVE DATA
INTRAPARTUM FETAL tpH MONITORING

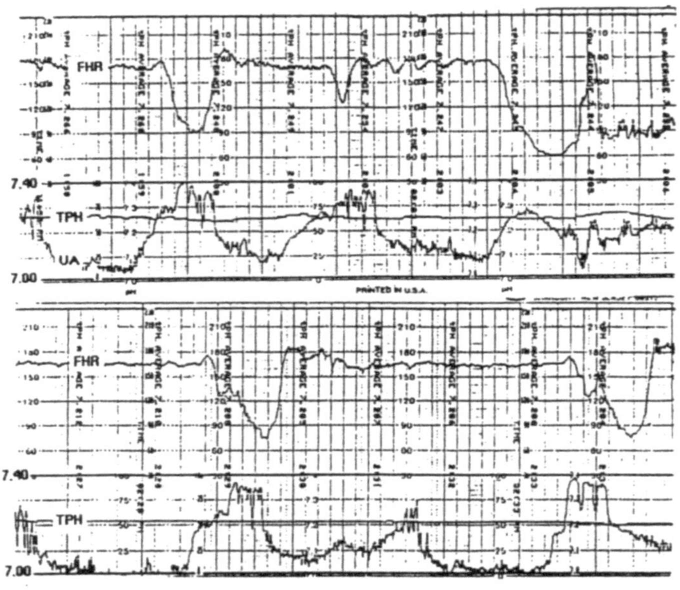

Figure 5 **Chart Display of Simultaneous Fetal Monitor and OBpH Data**

The fetal heart rate (FHR) demonstrates significant decelerations concordant with uterine activity (UA). The UA channel includes a tpH scale which ranges from pH 7.00 (bottom of record) to 7.40 (top of UA channel). The tpH is displayed as a linear graph on the UA channel, and it is updated every 20 seconds with the average tpH for the past 20 seconds. Each minute the average tpH is printed on the FHR channel (vertical printed statements). The FetaScan video displays the 20 second updated tpH value.

In-Vitro Performance of the OBpH System

In order to be useful as a trend monitor the OBpH system must resolve changes in pH at least as well as the current technology: the BpH. The 95% confidence interval (ci) of the BpH measurement is reported to be 0.06 pH or greater, with a non-Gaussian distribution (13,14). In-vitro studies of the OBpH probe demonstrate the 95% ci is 0.03 pH (Fig. 6). The absolute accuracy is within ±0.05 pH of a blood gas analyzer, which is also within the 95% confidence limits of blood measurement. Published data (8,15) show the high degree of correlation R>0.9 with in-vitro measurements of human fetal and adult blood.

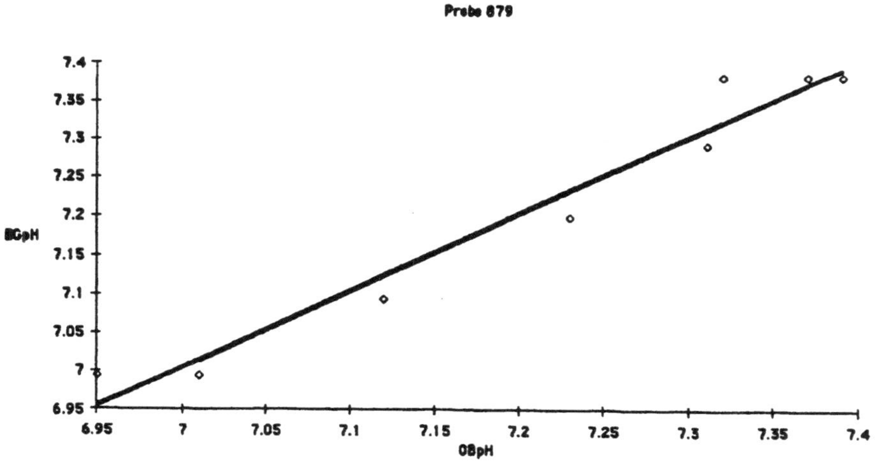

Figure 6 **Reproducibility of pH Measurement with a Single Fiberoptic tpH Probe**

The OBpH 1500 data is compared to blood gas analyzer pH (BGpH) at eight data points. The probe is first calibrated and then immersed in buffers of six other pH, and it is recycled through all eight pH at least twice. The probe must reproduce each data point within a bandwidth of ±0.03pH.

Clinical Investigational Plan

The feasibility model 1000 OBpH system was used in eight U.S. centers to monitor over 300 term or post-date high risk patients where BpH was indicated. The BpH was used to document the reliability of the current technology, the BpH, in following trends and to validate the reliability and the OBpH monitor in following trends of fetal pH status and in classifying fetal pH status as normal vs. not-normal.

The study goals:

1. Document the incidence of fetal or maternal problems caused by the OBpH in order to compare its safety with current technology.
2. Measure the *inherent* reliability of the tpH data for monitoring fetal pH status. "Inherent" means both the BpH and the OBpH data were unflawed or untainted, according to the investigator's report and an independent non-clinician reviewer at International Biomedics.
3. Document the perceived added value and clinical relevance of the OBpH monitoring data, when used as an adjunct to EFM and BpH measurements.

Clinical Study Methods

- Subject selection criteria:
  - Term or post-date patients in labor with vertex fetal presentation, and sufficient dilation and station to properly place the probe.
  - A documented indication for fetal scalp blood sampling for pH measurements.
  - No contraindications to fetal scalp blood sampling for pH measurements.
  - Informed consent given.

- Study Population: (Table I)

TABLE I
Study Population

	OBpH 1000	OBpH 1500
Total Patients	296	30
Total Formal Reports	291	30
Average Maternal Age	25 years	25 years
Average Gestational Age	39.9 wks	40.5 wks
Average Duration of OBpH Monitoring	2.0 hours	2:23 hours
Indications for pH Monitoring (% Cases)		
Abnormal FHR	83%	39%
Meconium	32%	28%
Post-date	21%	40%
Hypertension	16%	4%?
Diabetes	6%	---
Other	46%	36%
Pertinent Medications (% Cases)		
Oxytocin	42%	27%
Magnesium Sulfate	12%	-0-
Tocolytics	3%	-0-
Mode of Delivery (% Cases)		
Spontaneous Vaginal	61%	83%
Cesarean section	26%	17%
Forceps	11%	-0-
Vacuum	1%	-0-
No data	1%	-0-

TABLE I (CON)
Study Population

	OBpH 1000	OBpH 1500
Neonatal Problems		
Nuchal cord	9%	10%
Respiratory difficulties	3%	3%
Meconium aspiration	3%	-0-
Other	7%	-0-
One Minute Apgar Scores		
- 3	6%	-0-
4-6	18%	-0-
7-10	78%	100%
Adverse Effects	3.8%	-0-

• "Qualified Data Analysis" was used to measure the intrinsic reliability of the OBpH to monitor (correlate with) fetal CpH measurements, given no experimental flaws or "tainted data" and given the inherent variability of the CpH data. The correlation of replicate fetal CpH measures was determined in order to quantify the reliability of the current technology. Next, the tpH-CpH correlation data were calculated for those data points with replicate CpH, and then for all qualified sets of related tpH-CpH (Table II).

• "Physiological Data Analysis" was used to measure the clinical reliability of OBpH in trending fetal pH status, as measured by the correlation coefficient, given no obvious problems known to the investigator and pH values in the system operating range 7.09-7.44. (Tables II & III).

• Reliability of classification of fetal CpH by the OBpH data. These data included the predictive value of a normal tpH (7.20-7.44) vs. a normal CpH (7.25+) and the accuracy of both normal and not normal tpH to respectively predict normal & not normal CpH (efficiency of tpH). These data quantified the reliance the clinician can place as the tpH reflecting the CpH status. (Tables II & III).

• Success in obtaining a reliable OBpH trend record as compared to the success of obtaining reliable CpH measurements was measured. Certain conditions are known to interfere with blood pH and fetal scalp ECG reliability because free access to the scalp is blocked, and these similarly interfere with OBpH probe fixation. The most notable in this study was thick matted fetal hair. Meconium, scalp edema and duration of monitoring or labor did not consistently interfere with OBpH or BpH data.

• The potential clinical relevance of the OBpH data in patient management in addition to the FHR and BpH data was reported on the data forms and tallied.

TABLE II

Reliability of the OBpH 1000 Data (Feasibility Model)

	Correlation Coefficients: Weighted Mean	Correlation Coefficients: Range (among Institutions)
Total Case Reports with CpH and OBpH Data	198	
Qualified Data		
BpH/BpH: Blood pH reliability: (excluding Corometrics 220 Analyzer CpH data)	r=0.81	r=0.71-0.90
OBpH/BpH (Trending reliability):	r=0.84	r=0.72-0.94

Reliability of Classification of BpH by OBpH 1000 Data

Unflawed Physiological Data:	n=213 pairs.
Predictive Value of Normal tpH:	100%
False normal tpH:	0%
Efficiency (correct class./total):	68%

TABLE III
Reliability of the OBpH 1500 Data

Total Case Reports with both CpH and OBpH Data	20 (2 institutions)	
	Correlation Coefficients	
	Weighted Mean	Range
Physiological Data		
BpH/BpH: Blood pH reliability:	Insufficient Data	
OBpH/BpH:	r=0.89	r=0.79-0.93

Reliability of Classification of BpH by OBpH 1500 Data

Unflawed Physiological Data:	n=20 pairs
Predictive Value of Normal tpH:	100%
False Normal OBpH:	-0-
Efficiency (correct class/total):	89%

Success in Obtaining Fetal pH Data

The clinical experience demonstrated a continuous OBpH monitoring record could be obtained as frequently as a single valid fetal scalp blood pH data point (80%). With the OBpH 1500, the process was perceived to be simpler than obtaining one set of fetal scalp blood pH data point.

Clinical Relevance of the OBpH Data

The OBpH data was perceived as clinically relevant in 65% of these case reports. The most commonly mentioned advantages were:

•Reassurance of fetal pH stability and normalcy, especially despite other changes suggestive of possible fetal deterioration. (Abnormal FHR, Thick Meconium) This impression was validated by the 100% predictive value of a normal tpH.

•**Avoiding extra fetal scalp blood samples.**

•**Detecting trends in pH before they can be resolved by the blood pH method.** (Because of the OBpH self consistency)

•**Using the OBpH record as a guide to timing fetal scalp sampling for blood pH.** Usually there is no clear-cut indication as to when the pH is changing and may need diagnostic confirmation. The OBpH trend uniquely provides this information.

•**Monitoring fetal pH status where it is impractical to obtain timely repetitive blood pH data.** This is particularly relevant during stage II of labor, when abnormal heart rate patterns are common.

Discussion and Conclusions

The data demonstrated the OBpH system and the tpH method was inherently capable of reliable monitoring of fetal pH status, albeit with a different absolute value. The inherent consistency of the OBpH was obscured by the variability of the current technology, the BpH, the additional inter-institutional difference in BpH reliability; and possibly by clinical factors such as thick fetal hair. Also, there is an initial learning curve effect. At the start of the program, the correlation coefficient of tpH to OBpH was about 0.6. The last studies revealed correlation coefficients of 0.8 to 0.95 with a few or no tainted data points. Throughout the study, there were no false normal tpH values. When the tpH was 7.25 to 7.44, the unflawed BpH was always in the normal range.

Most clinicians perceived the data from the OBpH system to be clinically relevant, especially in monitoring trends of fetal pH status during worrisome events or events where repetitive timely BpH cannot be obtained. The investigators also immediately perceived the reliability of a normal and stable OBpH record.

To date, the clinical results obtained from the OBpH 1500 system are encouraging with respect to both practicality and reliability of the data.

References

(1) Anonymous: Antenatal Diagnosis. NIH Concensus Development Conference. March 5-7, 1979. US Dept HEW PHS NIH. NIH Publication No 79 (1973)

(2) Young DC, JH Gray, ER Luther et al: Fetal scalp blood pH sampling: Its value in an active obstetric unit. Am J Obstet Gynecol 126 (1980) 276

(3) Van den Berg P, S Schmidt, J Gesche, E Saling: Fetal distress and the condition of the newborn using cardiotocography and fetal blood analysis during labour. Brit J Obstet Gynaecol 94 (1987) 72

(4) Lagercrantz H, TA Soltkin: The "stress" of being born. Scientific American 254 4 (Apr. 1986) 100

(5) ACOG: ACOG Technical Bulletin 42 (1976): Fetal blood sampling.

(6) Stamm O, U Latscha, P Janacek, A Campana: Kontinuierliche pH-Messung am kindlichen Kopf post partum und sub partu und post partum (Continuous subcutaneaous assy of pH on the head of the infant after and during delivery). Z Geburtshilfe Perinatol. 178 (1974) 368

(7) Stamm O, P Janacek, A Campana: Registro continuo del pH tissular en perinatologia. Acta Ginecologica 26 (1975) 165

(8) Chatterjee M, F Hetzel, A Kaminetzky: Fetal tissue pH - Continuous intrapartum monitoring. Int J Gynaecol Obstet 22 (1984) 41

(9) Weber T: pH monitoring during labour with special reference to continuous fetal scalp tissue pH. Danish Medical Bulletin 30 (1983) 215

(10) Lauersen NH, FC Miller, RH Paul: Evaluation of continuous fetal scalp pH during labor. Arch Gynecol 226 (1978) 141

(11) Kellner KR, TC Key, AC Cruz, WN Spellacy: Evaluation of a continuous tissue pH monitor in the human fetus during labor. Obstet Gynecol 55 (1980) 523

(12) Flynn AM, J Kelly: The continuous measurement of tissue pH on the human fetus during labour using a new application technique. Br J Obstet Gynaecol 87 (1980) 666

(13) Lumley J et al: The unreliability of a single estimation of fetal scalp blood pH. J Lab Clin Med 77 (1971) 535

(14) Renou P, C Wood, J Lumley: Intrapartum fetal monitoring. In: Laurensen NH (ed.) "Modern Management of High Risk Pregnancy". Plenum, New York 1983

(15) Suidan JS, BK Young, FW Hetzel et al: pH measurement with a fiberoptic tissue-pH monitor and a standard blood-pH meter. Clinical Chemistry 29 (1983) 1566

(16) Roby PV, HM Hochberg, HE Fox et al: OBpH 1000 fetal tissue pH monitor clinical trial, Abst AAMI, Los Angeles 1987

ANIMAL STUDIES FOR INTRAPARTUM BIOCHEMICAL MONITORING - ARTIFICIAL UMBILICAL CIRCULATION

S. Schmidt

Department of Obstetrics & Gynecology, University of Bonn,
Sigmund-Freud-Straße 25, D-5300 Bonn, FRG

The electrode for the measurement of the transcutaneous partial pressure of carbon dioxide ($tcPCO_2$) is an additional instrument for the supervision of the fetus during labour (5,9,12). The investigation of certain aspects of the $tcPCO_2$ monitoring in the human fetus during labour was performed during a number of animal experiments in order to study the electrode under defined conditions.

The study of the response of electrochemical sensors have been shown to be limited during clinical trials to some extent (13). The aim of this paper is to demonstrate the reliability of a combined $tcPCO_2/PCO_2$ sensor to measure the PCO_2 and PO_2 in arterial blood over a wide range of values. The variability of the gases was achieved by an artificial umbilical circulation via a membranlung (1,2,7,11).

Method

The animal experiments were performed using twelve premature lambs, gestational age 125 to 128 days of gestation (caesarian section in epidural anesthesia). The delivered premature lambs directyl thereafter were connected to a perfusion circuit using catheters that were implanted into the umbilical artery and umbilical vein (thinwalled, largewalled catheters embedding stainless steel springs (14). The perfusion circuit included an 0,4 m Scimed - Kolobow membrane lung, 3/16 Polyurethan-tubing and a mechanical pump. The priming volume of 160 ml was maternal blood. The flow rate in the extracorporeal circuit was initially regulated aiming at a PCO_2 of 45 to 55 mm HG. PCO_2 values in the extracorporeal circuit were measured by intermitten blood samples from the arterial line and by a sensor and a flow chamber that measured the PCO_2 and PO_2 values at a measuring temperature of 37 °C. The circuit and the animal were thermostated at 37°C by means of an incubator. Transcutaneous electrodes were placed on the fetal head by the glue technique (4). The measuring site was prepared in the following way: hair was removed and the measuring site was cleansed from mucus and blood using squabs. Fixation rings thereafter were applied on this measuring site using butylcyanoacrylat. The rings were then filled with contact solution and the electrode was screwed into the fixation rings. On an schematic drawing the experimental set up that is used during the investigation is demonstrated (Fig. 1).

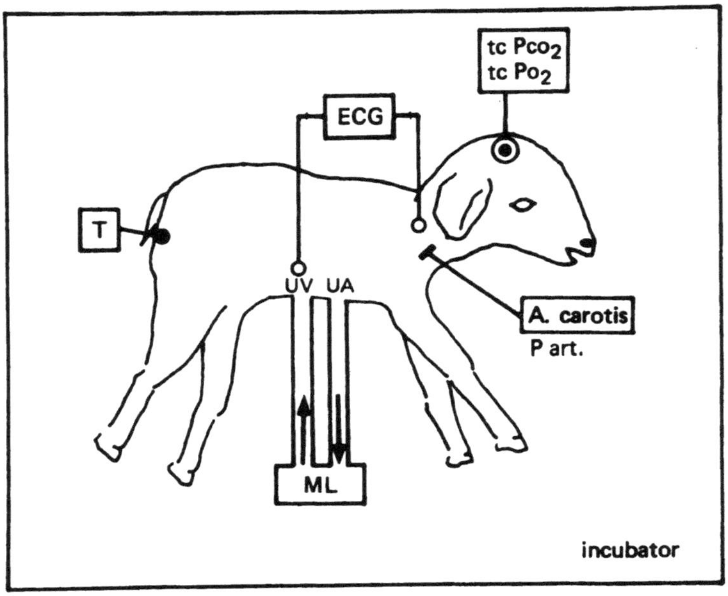

Fig. 1 Schematic drawing of the experimental set up: premature lamb connected via the umbilical vessels (UV,UA) to an extra corporeal arteriovenous circuit to a membrane lung (ML) - Blood pressure (P.art) temperature (T) and heart frequency (ECG) are monitored. $TcPCO_2$ and $tcPO_2$ is continously recorded.

The data of the continuously recorded PCO_2 measurement using the transcutaneous technique was compared with the results of blood gas checks of blood samples taken from the arteria carotis. The arterial blood pressure was recorded continuously (A. carotis) by means of a Statham system.

The experimental set up of an artificial umbilical circulation with a connection to membrane lung that provides a CO_2 removal and oxygenation enables to study the PCO_2 and PO_2 and its registration by transcutaneous electrodes over a wide range of gas values at different flow rates in the umbilical circuit and different gas concentration in the membrane lung. On the multi-channel-recorder the data of the transcutaneous tracings of PCO_2 and PO_2 as recorded by the Draeger electrodes at 44°C as well as the recorded arterial blood pressure as well as the heartrate of the lamb (Fig. 2).

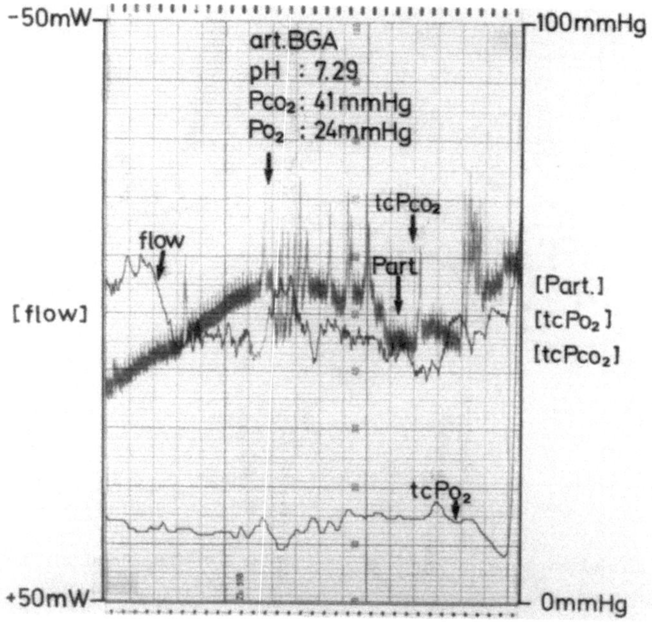

Fig. 2 Registration of Part, $tcPCO_2$ and $tcPO_2$ and the heart rate and relative heat deviation (flow) as well as the result of intermittend blood gas analysis (BGA) during artificial umbilical circulation.

Results

The comparison between the transcutaneous PCO_2 -values and the values in the fetal blood as collected during the experiments clearly shows a characteristic overestimation of the PCO_2 by the transcutaneous system. This overestimation occurs characteristicly during transcutaneous recordings of PCO_2 due to the raised temperature and CO_2 production in the tissue. There was a statistically significant correlation ($r = 0{,}91$ $p < 0{,}0001$). While the intecept was 17,80 and the slope 0,99 (Fig. 3).

For the comparison between $tcPO_2$ and PO_2 values we also found a good correlation ($r = 0{,}89$). There was a tendence to underestimate the gas value in the blood though (intercept=-10,36).

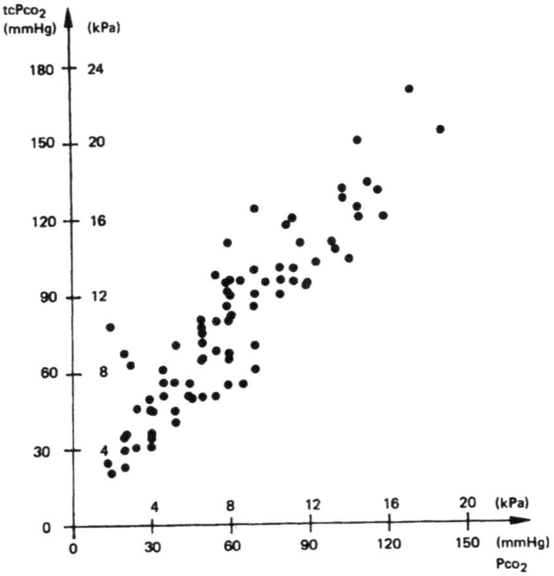

Fig. 3 Correlation between $tcPCO_2$ and PCO_2 in the blood of the premature lamb (r=o,91, p <0,00001, intercept =+ 17,80, slope = 0,99).

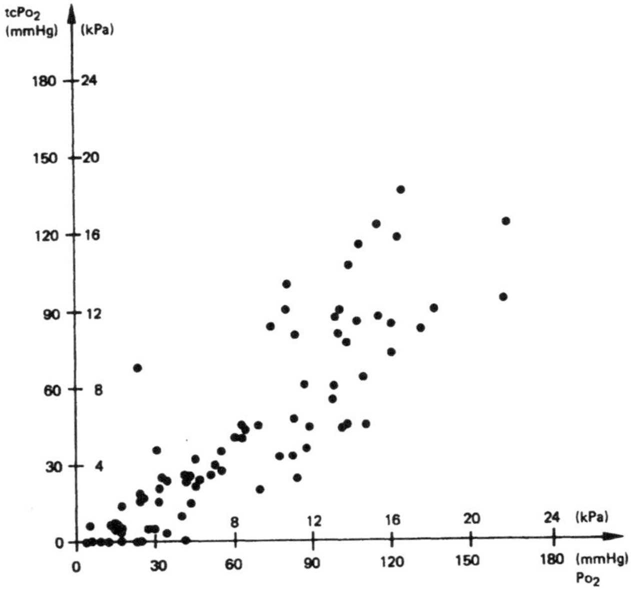

Fig. 4 Correlation between $tcPO_2$ and PO_2 (r=0,89, p< 0,00001, intercept = - 10,37, slope = 0,80).

Discussion

Two different experimental set ups have been described before for the study of tc-sensors. The Rudolph-technique - chronically instrumented sheep - has the advantage that using the original technique animals can be investigated in a steady state situation (6,7,8,14). When investigating transcutaneous electrodes one has the disadvantage of the fact that the electrodes ideally should be implanted during the first session and then would have to be fixed on the fetal head by head by a technique that garanties that a dislodging does not occur (3,4,5,13). While basically an in vivo calibration of the electrode would be possible I would suspect that a dislodging of the electrode using a glue technique is very likely after a period of five days. On the other hand, if no leakage occurs one would be afraid of changes in the perfusion of the skin below the electrode leading to edema of the skin. If the animal experiments with chronically catheterized animals are performed using a second laparotomy, one has to keep in mind that during the second laparotomy it is again possible to cause a considerable disturbance of the fetal circulation (8,10). In this sense the data collected during our experiments can only to some extend be interpreted as data of a chronical experiment (8,10).
Using the technique of artificial umbilical circulation one has the advantage that using a membrane lung it is possible to change the PCO_2 and PO_2 values in the fetal blood over a large range. Additionally using a PCO_2 and PO_2 -flow-probe it is possible to compare the data with a transcutaneous data synchronously and continuously. On the other hand it is a disadvantage of this technique that the environment even if using an incubator is different from an intrauterine situation which leads to a larger oxygen up-take and additionally if the necessity of ventilation occurs it induces a disturbance of the fetal circulation (10). In this way data collected during such experiments can only to a certain degree be compared with the biological intrauterine situation. The problematic of such an experiments can only to a certain degree be compared with the biological intrauterine situation. The problematic of such an experiment is also very well demonstrated by the fact that a transcutaneous to fetal blood difference for PO_2 even data are corrected of occur during such experiments, that shows very clearly that a certain amount of a centralisation leading to a disturbance in the skin perfusion can be detected which is shown on the last Figure. Such disturbance occurs during the first hours of such a perfusion and is only improved after some three hours (unpublished observation). In conclusion we might say that animal experiments lead to the possibility of investigation of transcutaneous trancings of PCO_2 and PO_2 under defined conditions. A clerification of certain aspects is achieved. None of the

experimental set ups used by our group ideally simulate the fetal environment and one should additionally keep in mind that certain aspects such as compression phenomena that occur rhythmically during the fetal measurment in the human as well as the phenomenon of the diffusion disturbance during caput succedaneum may not very well be simulated during such animal experiments so that the influence of such circumstances occuring with the progress of labour should be inbestigated only during clinical trials (4,12,13).

References

(1) Bartels H, W Moll: Passage of inert substances and oxygen in the human placenta. Pflügers Arch ges Physiol 280 (1965) 165

(2) Bradley AF, M Stupfel, JW Severinghaus: Effect of temperature on PCO_2 and PO_2 of blood in vitro. J Appl Physiol 9 (1956) 201

(3) Huch A, R Huch, K Meinzer, DW Lübbers: Eine schnelle, beheizte pt-Oberflächenelektrode zur kontinuierlichen Überwachung des PO_2 beim Menschen. Elektrodenaufbau und Eigenschaften. Medizintechnik (1972) 26

(4) Huch A, R Huch: Klinische und physiologische Aspekte der transkutanen Sauerstoffdruckmessung in der Perinatalmedizin. Z Geburtsh u Perinatal 179 (1975) 235

(5) Huch R, A Huch: Continuous PO_2 and PCO_2 monitoring in the neonate. J Perinat Med 9 (1981) 200

(6) Jansen CAM, FG Bass, KC Lowe, PW Nathanielsz: Comparison of continuous transcutaneous and continous intravascular PO_2 measurement in fetal sheep. Am J Obstet Gynecol 138 (1980) 670

(7) Jensen A, W Künzel: The difference between fetal transcutaneous PO_2 and arterial PO_2 during labour. Gynecol Obstet Invest 11 (1980) 249

(8) Künzel W, E Kastendieck, CS Kurz: A comparative study of continuous intra vascular O_2 saturation and transcutaneous PO_2 measurements in the sheep fetus following the reduction of uterine blood flow. In: Huch, Huch, Lucey (eds.): 1st International Symposium on Continuous Transcutaneous Blood Gas Monitoring, Marburg 1978. The National Foundation of Birth Defects. Original Article Series, Liss, New York 1979

(9) Lübbers DW, U Grossmann: Gas exchange through the human epidermis as a basis of $tcPO_2$ and $tcPCO_2$ measurement. In: Huch R, A Huch (eds.): Continuous transcutaneous blood gas monitoring. Marcel Dekker, Inc, New York, Basel 1983

(10) Rudolf AM, MA Heymann, Methods for studying the circulation of the fetus in utero.: In: Nathanielsz PW (ed.): Animal models in fetal medicine, Elsevier-North-Holland-Biochemical Press, Amsterdam 1980

(11) Saling E: Neues Vorgehen zur Untersuchung des Kindes unter der Geburt. Einführung, Technik und Grundlagen. Arch Gynäk 197 (1962) 108

(12) Schmidt S, K Langner, J Rothe, E Saling: A new combined electrode for $tcPCO_2$-measurement and fetal heart rate recording. J Perinat Med 10 (1982) 297

(13) Schmidt S, K Langner, J Gesche, JW Dudenhausen, E Saling: Der transkutan gemessene Kohlendioxydpartialdruck beim nichthypoxischen Feten während der Geburt. Geburtsh u Frauenheilk 43 (1983) 538
(14) Schmidt S, K Langner, CH Laiblin, JW Dudenhausen, J Gesche, E Saling: Response time of the $tcPCO_2$ electrode - an animal experimental study. Biomed Technik 29 (1984) 289
(15) Severinghaus JW, M Stafford, AF Bradley: $tcPCO_2$ electrode design, calibration and temperature gradient problems. Acta anaesth scand 68 (1978) 118

METHODOLOGY AND CLINICAL VALUE OF TRANSCUTANEOUS BLOOD GAS MEASUREMENTS IN THE FETUS

S. Schmidt

Departement of Obstetrics & Gynecology, University of Bonn,
Sigmund-Freud-Straße 25, D-5300 Bonn, FRG

Summary

Aiming at an improvement of fetal surveillance in high risk cases, a clinical trial was performed to evaluate the potential of fetal $tcPco_2$ monitoring. An electrochemical $tcPco_2$ sensor heated at 44 °C was applied in 119 fetuses after abnormal heart rate patterns had occured. The number of operative deliveries for fetal distress was reduced to 14 cases by means of the biochemical parameters ($tcPco_2$) and fetal blood analysis (FBA). In the majority of cases with pathologic heart rate patterns the $tcPco_2$ values were prepathologic or normal (60 %), while in 68 % of cases with prepathologic heart rate patterns the $tcPco_2$ level was normal. At all instances an intrauterine complication was indicated by a marked rise of the $tcPco_2$ level. The clinical benefit of using the $tcPco_2$ measurement is the better specificity of detecting fetal distress when compared with the use of cardiotocography alone. Furthermore the $tcPco_2$ technique has the advantage of providing continuous information about one biochemical parameter and of avoiding the necess ity of repeated incisions of the scalp, as compared with the technique of fetal blood analysis. In conclusion the use of this non-traumatic technique lends itself to avoid unnecessary operative deliveries in high risk cases.

Keywords: fetal monitoring, transcutaneous measurement, FBA, $tcPco_2$, CTG, fetal distress.

Fetal heart rate monitoring, which is used by the large majority of obstetricians, is of high value as a screening method as it has a high sensitivity but provides a number of false positive results (2,11). By indicating fetal distress which does not acutally exist, it leads to unnecessary operative deliveries, when used as the only method of fetal surveillance. It was the aim of this study to evaluate the potential clinical benefit of the $tcPco_2$-monitoring during labor, which provides reliable information about one biochemical parameter in the fetus during labour, to verify fetal distress in cases where an intrauterine complication is indicated by abnormal fetal heart rate patterns (8, 10).

Material and methods

During the course of this study $tcPco_2$ -measurements were performed in 119 fetuses in addition to continuous cardiotocography. Cases were included in the study when either suspect, prepathologic or pathologic heart rate patterns occured in the CTG on admission or during labour. Fetal blood analysis (FBA) was performed when the following cardiotocographic changes were observed: decelerations-variable, late, early (more than 60 bpm) - for more than 10 minutes or 3 contractions, and immediately in cases with severe bradycardia (less than 100 bpm). 85 mothers were para 0, 13 were para I, 21 were para II or more. The patients were given detailed information about the $tcPco_2$ -measurement and informed consent was achieved. 76 infants were born spontaneously, 15 by vacuum extraction, 5 with the help of modified forceps. In 23 cases cesarean section had to be performed.

Operative delivery for fetal distress was performed in 14 cases. The indication for an operative delivery for fetal distress was based on the heart rate pattern, the level of the $tcPco_2$ and the result of the FBA.

The status of the newborns was evaluated with a modified Apgar Score in combination with a biochemical analysis of a sample from the umbilical artery (5). All babies were born in vigorous state ($\geqslant$ 7). As the result of pH-measurements in umbilical artery blood (samples collected directly after delivery), we found a value of below 7.20 in 8 cases, a value of 7.20 - 7.29 in 26 cases, while in the rest of the 86 cases, the pH-values were $\geqslant$ 7.30.

The $tcPco_2$ -measurement was performed using the modified Severinghaus electrode (Radiometer B 5230), the details of which have been described elsewhere (7, 10). After sterilisation and a two-point-calibration, the electrode was applied onto the fetal scalp and fixed by means of tissue glue. The measuring temperature for this trial was 44° in all cases. Transcutaneous Pco_2 -values were not corrected for the metabolism of the skin and the raised local tissue temperature. The maximal drift which was evaluated by means of a calibration gas was 2 %. The results of the $tcPco_2$ -measurements were entered on the enquiry form together with the findings of the vaginal examination, the result of the concurrent fetal blood analysis, the result of the evaluation of the retrograde cardiotocogram (Hammacher-Score) and the indication for fetal blood analysis (1). Data were fed into a Cyber 70 (Control Data) and evaluated with the Statistic

Package for Social Science (SPSS) of Northwestern University. The linear correlation coefficient, the slope, the intercept and the significance were calculated for the comparison of continuous $tcPco_2$ levels to the blood analysis (FBA) and the pH. In order to plot the mean $tcPco_2$ of the second stage of labour the transcutaneous measurement was scanned at a sampling frequency of ten minutes and compared with the result of the assessment of the newborn. Furthermore, in order to investigate the statistical relationship between the measuring data of the $tcPco_2$ and the result of the semiquantitative evaluation of the Hammacher-Score, the contigency coefficients according to Pearson were calculated. As a basis for this calculation a table of nine fields was drawn up for the chi-square test. The result of the Hammacher-Score (HS) respectively the transcutaneously measured carbon-dioxide-partial-pressure were defined as normal (HS=0-2 respectively $tcPco_2 \leqslant 70$ mmHg), prepathologic (HS=3-7 respectively $tcPco_2 > 70$-80 mmHg and pathologic ($HS \geqslant 8$ respectively $tcPco_2 > 80$ mmHg).

Results

The accuracy ot the $tcPco_2$ technique to measure the Pco_2 of the blood was approved by comparing the Pco_2 values of the fetal blood analysis with the synchronously recorded $tcPco_2$. We found a statistically significant relationship ($r = 0.81$, $p < 0.001$) (Fig. 1). Furthermore the transcutaneous Pco_2 values recorded at the moment of delivery correlated with the Pco_2 values of the umbilical artery ($r = 0{,}76$; $p < 0{,}001$ (Fig 2)). In order to define the prepathologic and pathologic range of $tcPco_2$ we evaluated the relationship between $tcPco_2$ and pH values in the fetal blood (8). The actual pH value was compared with the synchronously recorded $tcPco_2$ value. We found a statistically significant correlation ($p < 0.001$). The correlation coefficient for 44°C was -0.53, the intercept 788.83 and there was a negative slope of -0.99. While there was a considerable scattering of $tcPco_2$ values in the pH range of above 7.25, no preacidosis occured during $tcPco_2$ values of < 70 mmHg and no pH values of < 7.20 were observed with $tcPco_2$ values of < 80 mmHg at 44 ° C. The mean value of the transcutaneous measurement during the second stage of labour was compared with the result of the assessment of the newborn. The $tcPco_2$ level was significantly lower in normacidic newborns when compared with the $tcPco_2$ level in cases with raised acidity respectively acidosis ($2a = o0{,}05$) (Fig. 3). Comparing the $tcPco_2$ values with the results of clinical assessment we found that the mean value of cases with an Apgar score of 10 was significantly lower as with an Apgar score of 9 respectively 8 ($2a = 0{,}05$), (Kruskall-Wallis-Test) (Fig. 4). With the use of a multi-channel-recorder it was possible to provide a continuous poly-

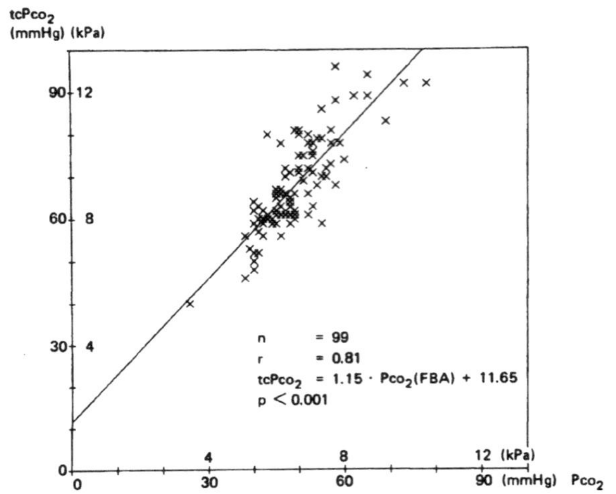

Fig. 1 Correlation between the transcutaneously measured carbon-dioxide-partial-pressure ($tcPco_2$) and the Pco_2 of the fetal blood analysis (FBA): The $tcPco_2$ values measured at 44° are not corrected for the effect of raised temperature nor the Co_2 production of the tissue.

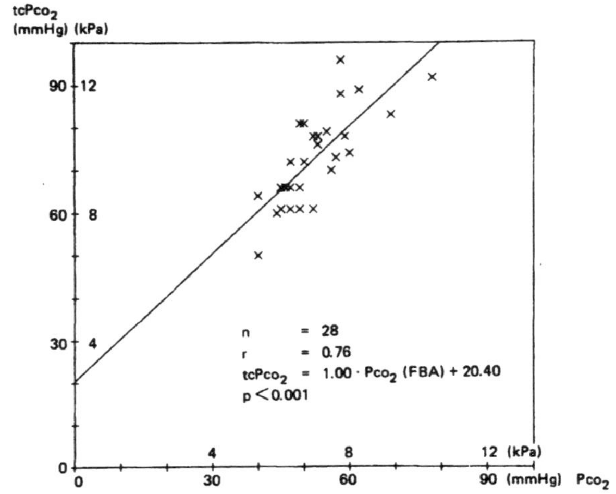

Fig. 2 Correlation between the $tcPco_2$ at the moment of delivery and the Pco_2 measured in a blood sample of the umbilical artery (UA).

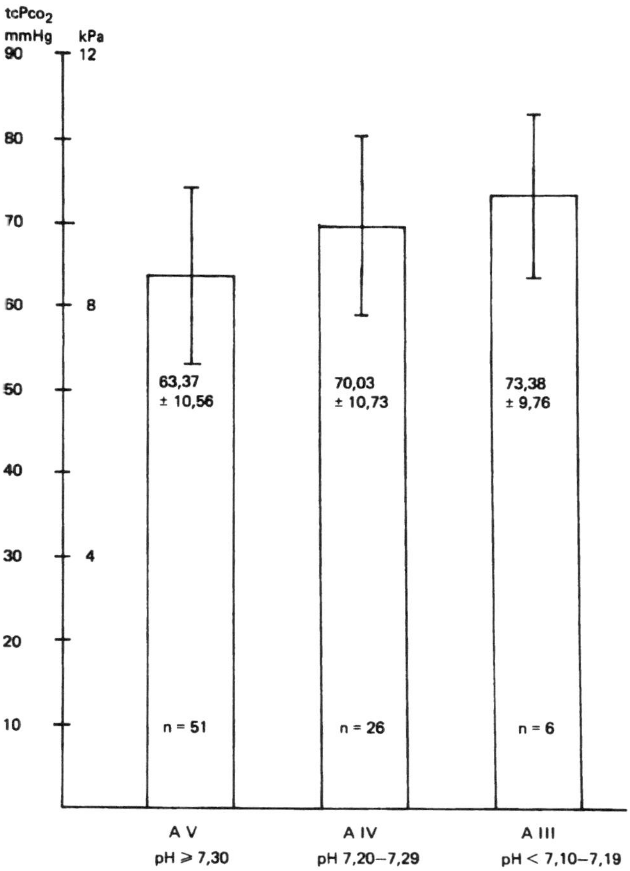

Fig. 3 Mean value and standard deviation of the $tcPco_2$ during the second stage of labour according to the result of the biochemical assessment of the newborn (pH in umbilical artery blood).

graphic recording of both the cardiotocogram and the data of the transcutaneous measurement. Various combinations of heart rate patterns and the level of the transcutaneous Pco_2 were observed (see Fig. 5-7). A suspicious CTG in combination with a normal level of the $tcPco_2$ can be seen in the tracing with the registration number 39/44. During the first stage of labour variable decelerations were observed in the CTG; however the $tcPco_2$ was within the normal range. There was no indication for operative delivery for fetal distress superfluous in this case. After spontaneous delivery the baby was vigorous and normacidic (pH in the umbilical artery 7,25).

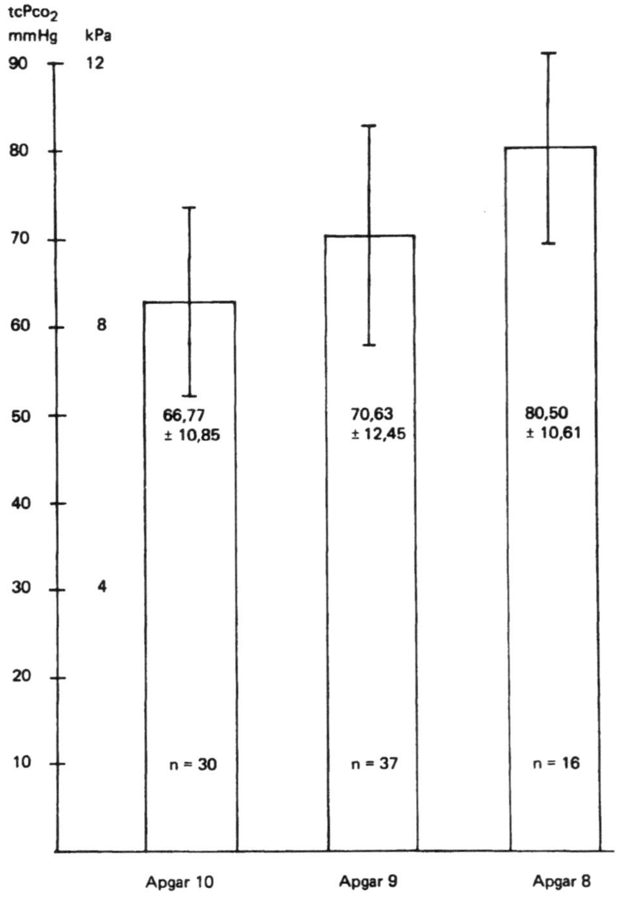

Fig. 4 Mean value and standard deviation of the $tcPco_2$ during the second stage of labour according to the results of the clinical assessment of the newborn (modified Apgar score).

A critical rise of the $tcPco_2$ during pathologic heart rate pattern is demonstrated on Fig. 6 with the registration number 11/44. The baby was born by immediate cesarean section after the intrauterine complication had been verified by FBA. Due to the clear indication of fetal distress by means of the $tcPco_2$ -tracing it was possible to perform the obstetrical intervention right on time. In spite of acidosis (pH UA $<$ 7,20), the baby was delivered before signs of clinical depression had been manifested. The polygraphic tracing shown in Fig. 7 (registration number 10/44) demonstrates how a fast progressing intrauterine complication

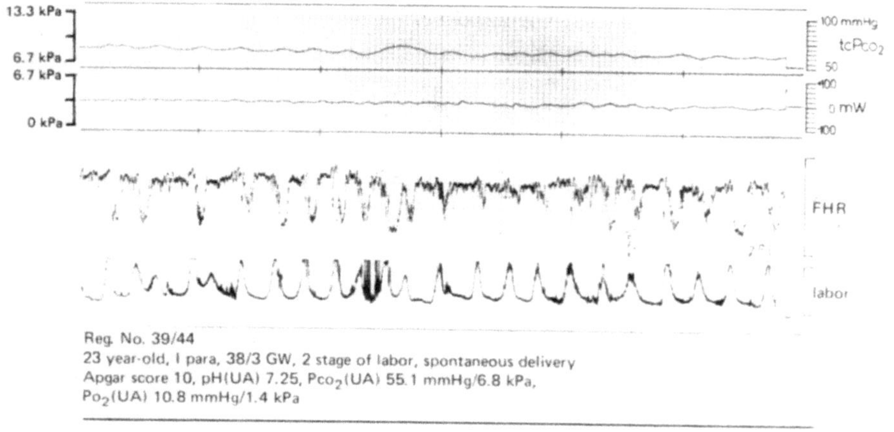

Fig. 5 Registration of tcP_{CO_2} (mmHg), relative heat deviation (mW), fetal heart rate (FHR) and labour in a case where, in spite of abnormal heart rate pattern the tcP_{CO_2} -level remained within the normal range.

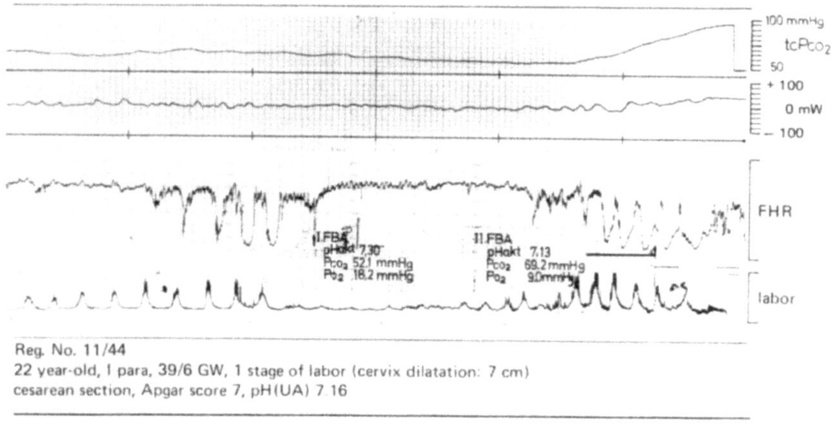

Fig. 6 Registration of tcP_{CO_2} (mmHg), relative heat deviation (mW), fetal heart rate (FHR) and labour. Whilst the abnormal heart rate pattern at the beginning of this registration is misleading as neither the tcP_{CO_2} values nor the values of the FBA I verify a disturbance, the moment of decompensation of the gas transfer is shown by a fast rise of tcP_{CO_2}. This complication was verified by fetal blood analysis (FBA II).

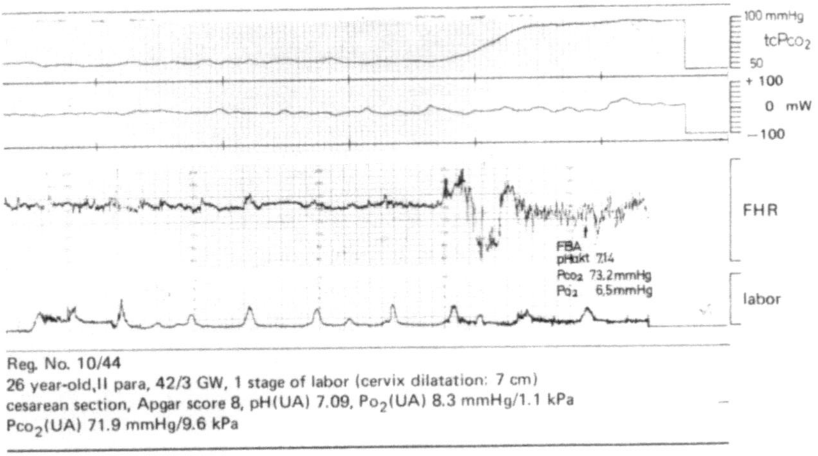

Fig. 7 Registration of $tcPco_2$ (mmHg), relative heat deviation (mW), fetal heart rate (FHR) and labour. In this case an acute intrauterine complication was more clearly indicated by the $tcPco_2$ -values than by the heart rate pattern.

H. -Score	44°C $tcPco_2$ (mmHg) ≤ 70	$> 70–80$	> 80
0–2	4		1
3–7	55	25	1
≥ 8	7	5	8

Fig. 8 Comparison between normal ($\leq$ 70 mmHg), prepathologic ($>$ 70-80) and pathologic ($>$ 80) $tcPco_2$ values and normal (0 - 2), prepathologic (3 - 7) and pathologic ($\geq$8) results of the Hammacher scoring system for the heart pattern (Hammacher 1974).

is more clearly indicated by the registration of the $tcPco_2$ than by the changes of the heart rate pattern. After an acceleration and a deceleration lasting only two and a half minutes, the heart rate returned to a normal value. The improved oscillation is additionally misleading, as it implicates a reestablished transplacental gas transfer. The continuous rise of the $tcPco_2$ level > 80 mmHg clearly indicates a progressing distrubance. After verifying the acidosis by means of a fetal blood analysis also this baby was born by immediate cesarean section without signs of clinical depression, though the pH had further decreased to a value of 7.09.

The conformity respectively the discrepancy of the two methods was evaluated statistically by means of the chi-square test (Fig. 8). The evalutation of 53 hours of synchronous registration had a level of 30,90 for the chi-square test. 0,48 was calculated as the contingency coefficient according to Pearson. The quantitative evaluation demonstrates the superior specificity of $tcPco_2$ to indicate fetal distress as compared with the cardiotocographic tracing. When the CTG was pathologic the $tcPco_2$ was prepathologic or even normal in 60 %. When the CTG was prepathologic the $tcPco_2$ -level was within the normal range in 68 % of the cases.

Discussion

A considerable reduction of perinatal mortality and morbidity has been achieved by modern clinical methods of fetal surveillance. In spite of this fact, the clinical benefit of electronic fetal monitoring is still controversial (4, 11). The enormous rise of operative deliveries for fetal distress as the result of the introduction of continous fetal monitoring is the major objection of some authors against the general application of this technique (2, 11). The indication of fetal distress in cases where actually no complication emerges is the major shortcoming of the CTG when used as the only technique of supervision (3) The complementary use of a biochemical parameter has been proposed as an adequate solution. The fetal blood analysis is a reliable method to identify an intrauterine complication (6). This technique has the disadvantage of only providing intermittent information about the biochemical status of the fetus, and in some cases has to be repeated at short intervals if fetal heart rate patterns remain pathological. Additionally a traumatisation of the fetal skin in inevitable, as an incision has to be made in order to take blood samples.

The transcutaneous measurement of carbon dioxide ($tcPco_2$) with a heated Severinghaus electrode in the fetus during labour provides reliable information about one biochemical parameter (8). There is a considerable scattering of $tcPco_2$ values when the Pco_2 of the blood is raised during a disturbance of the placental gas transfer. Such a phenomen can partly be explained by the fact that the electrochemical sensor traces the changes in the blood with considerable time lag and has been studied under defined condition in chronically instrumented pregnant sheep (9). By analysing the data of a clinical trial it was possible to define normal, prepathologic and pathologic values for the clinical use of the $tcPco_2$ in the fetus (8).

It should be mentioned that artefacts caused for example by a compression of the electrode or a caput succedaneum at the measuring site potentially result in raised $tcPco_2$ -levels in some cases (8). It thus seems to be advisable to confirm the intrauterine complication by the FBA technique. In this way it will also be possible to identify cases with only transient Pco_2 rise where no clinical intervention is necessary. Due to the good specificity of the $tcPco_2$ to indicate fetal distress it will be possible in the large majority of cases with suspicious, prepathologic and pathologic heart rate patterns to avoid unnecessary operative deliveries respectively the necessity to repreat fetal blood analysis. During this study the potential clinical benefit of the additional use of the $tcPco_2$ in cases where the cardiotocographic tracing indicated fetal distress was clearly approved. In spite of the fact that this clinical trial included cases with high risk of hypoxia, operative delivery for fetal distress was only performed in 12 % of the cases. On the other hand the $tcPco_2$ -recording informs and warns the obstetrician in the case of a disturbance of the gas transfer to the fetus occuring, even when the complication is not clearly indicated in the CTG. As the analysis of the data of this trial demonstrates, it will be possible to terminate labour early enough to avoid clinical manifestation of sub partu hypoxia. None of the babies of this trial were born in a clinically depressed state.

Hopefully the application of the $tcPco_2$ -electrode in the clinical surveillance of the fetus during labour will help to further improve the obstetrical management as it provides additional information in a non-traumatic and convenient way.

References

(1) Hammacher K, RB del Re, R Gaudenz, P De Grandi: Kardiotokographischer Nachweis einer fetalen Gefährdung mit einem CTG-Score. Gynäk Rdsch 14 (1974) 61

(2) Haverkamp AD, M Orleans, S Langendorfer, J McFee, J Murphy, HE Thomson: A controlled trial of the differential effects of intrapartum fetal monitoring. Am J Obstet Gynecol 134 (1979) 399

(3) Parer J: Benefits and detriments of fetal heart monitoring. Sem Perinat 2 (1978) 113

(4) Quilligan EJ, RH Paul: Fetal monitoring: is it worth it? Obstet Gynec 45 (1975) 96

(5) Saling E, KH Wulf: Zustandsdiagnostik beim Neugeborenen - Gruppeneinteilung. Fortsch Med 89 (1971) 12

(6) Saling E: Fetal scalp blood analysis. J Perinat Med 9 (1981) 165

(7) Schmidt S, K Langner, J Rothe, E Saling: A new combined non-invasive electrode for $tcPCO_2$-measurement and fetal heart rate recording. J Perinat Med 10 (1982) 297

(8) Schmidt S: Clinical trials on continuous measurement of fetal tcPCO. J Perinat Med 12 (1984) 241

(9) Schmidt S, K Langner, C Laiblin, JW Dudenhausen, J Gesche, E Saling: Ansprechzeit der tcPCO-Elektrode - eine tierexperimentelle Untersuchung. Biomed Tech 29 (1984) 289

(10) Severinghaus JW, M Stafford, AF Bradley: TcPCO electrode design, calibration and temperature gradient problems. Acta Anaesth Scand 68 (1978) 118

(11) Sykes GS, TM Molloy, P Johnson, JM Stirrat, AC Turnbull: Fetal distress and the condition of newborn infants. Br Med J 287 (1983) 943

CONTINUOUS TRANSCUTANEOUS CARBON DIOXIDE MONITORING DURING HUMAN LABOUR

C. Nickelsen
Department of Obstetrics and Gynecology, Rigshospitalet,
University of Copenhagen, Denmark

T. Weber
Department of Obstetrics and Gynecology, Hvidovre Hospital,
University of Copenhagen, Denmark

Introduction

Fetal transcutaneous carbon dioxide tension is the only possible method for non-invasive monitoring of the fetal acid base state during labour. During fetal respiratory acidosis the carbon dioxide tension is elevated. At least temporarily this is also found during fetal metabolic acidosis (1).

By the transcutaneous technique the gas tension of the extra cellular fluid in the upper layer of the skin is measured. This value reflects the gas tension of arterial blood but it is modified by the capillary blood flow and the production or consumption of gas in the area. Heating of the skin produces dilatation of the capillaries. This is necessary when transcutaneous oxygen is monitored. However, during transcutaneous carbon dioxide monitoring this is not quite as essential because of a much higher transmissibility of the carbon dioxide though the epidermal layers.

Heating of the skin - and the blood - will cause an elevation of the transcutaneous carbon dioxide tension in relation to the capillary value, which usually is measured at 37°C. The transcutaneous carbon dioxide tension should be corrected for this temperature difference. Additionally, the carbon dioxide production in the skin between the capillaries and the electrode on the skin surface will cause an elevation of the transcutaneous carbon dioxide tension. In previous studies this "metabolic" contribution to the transcutaneous carbon dioxide tension is estimated to be approximately 0.5 kPa (2).

The electrode used in our studies is a modified Severinghaus carbon dioxide electrode (Radiometer E 5230).

Sterilization implies change of electrode membrane, mechanical cleaning with alcohol and sterilization in fluid aldehydes. The electrode is calibrated at a 5% and 10% carbon dioxide gas mixture immediately before the final sterilization with aldehydes. No drift or change in electrode sensitivity has been observed during the final sterilization procedure (3).

Application of the electrode to the fetal scalp can be performed using either a glue fixation technique or a suction fixation technique. The glue fixation is performed through an amnioscope, using cotton swaps to clean and dry the fetal skin before applying the electrode with a specially designed forceps. In contrast, the suction fixation is performed without amnioscopy and without cleaning during a vaginal examination, holding the electrode in the suction ring between the two exploring fingers (Fig. 1). The electrode is kept in the position by a vacuum of 20

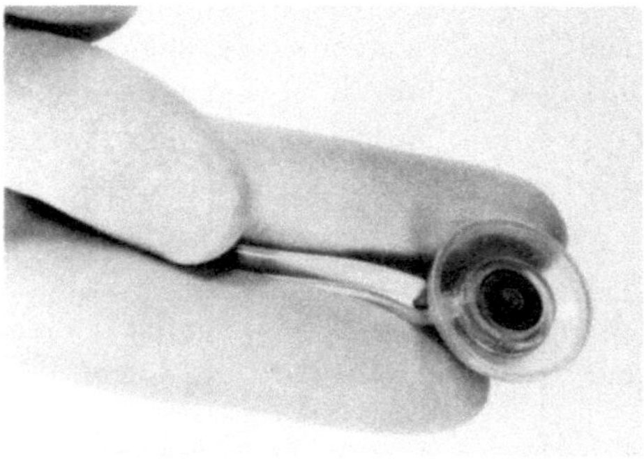

kPa produced by an electrical pump. We have compared the two methods by simultaneously monitoring a fetus with two electrodes applied by the two different methods (4). No difference in the measured carbon dioxide tension was found. Compression of the electrode on the other hand causes an elevation of the measured pCO_2. This was demonstrated in a study in which one electrode was placed under the cervical edge. This electrode measured higher tc-pCO_2 values which fluctuated with the uterine contraction compared to lower stable values measured by another electrode, which was not compressed (5). The suction fixation method makes it possible during a vaginal examination to move the electrode to a position without compression.

Results

We have performed monitoring with an electrode temperature of 44 °C (80 cases) and with an electrode temperature of 41°C (42 cases). When correlating the last measured transcutaneous carbon dioxide value just before delivery to the carbon dioxide tension of umbilical artery blood we found significant correlations using both electrode temperatures. The regression line was close to the identity line, but the intercept on the Y-axis was much higher when using the 41° C temperature than when using the 44°C temperature. This intercept is an indication of the mean difference between the umbilical artery blood value and the transcutaneous value. This could be explained by the lower temperature causing less dilatation of the capillaries of the skin and a subsequent lower blood flow and accumulation of carbon dioxide in the tissue.

The mean values of tc-pCO_2 are calculated according to the dilatation of the cervical os, slightly higher values being found using the low electrode temperature (Table 1). The values were slightly increasing during the first stage and more distinctly increasing during the second stage of labour.

During our studies only six newborns were delivered with umbilical artery blood pH below 7.15 following transcutaneous pCO2 monitoring. Using the above mentioned mean values + 2SD as upper limit for normal pCO2 only 4 out of these 6 newborns had values exceeding this limit. In all 6 cases there was a distinct increase of pCO2 before delivery.

Table 1. Mean $\pm$SD of fetal transcutaneous carbon dioxide tension according to the cervical dilatation, measured at different elecde temperatures.

	4 cm	5 cm	6 cm	7 cm	8 cm	9 cm	10 cm	PF
41°	6.16 $\pm$ 1.17	6.84 $\pm$ 1.67	7.07 $\pm$ 1.72	7.01 $\pm$ 1.42	7.15 $\pm$ 1.66	7.23 $\pm$ 1.40	7.33 $\pm$ 1.47	7.86 $\pm$ 2.06
n=	21	28	31	34	35	36	37	34
44°	5.82 $\pm$ 0.80	5.97 $\pm$ 0.75	6.01 $\pm$ 0.88	5.96 $\pm$ 0.89	6.18 $\pm$ 1.11	6.20 $\pm$ 1.05	6.37 $\pm$ 1.05	7.17 $\pm$ 1.13
n=	18	34	47	52	63	68	66	48

However, if all six acidotic fetuses (Umbilical artery pH $<$ 7.15) should be detected by a fixed tc-pCO2 limit the upper limit of tc-pCO2 should be as low as the mean value of tc-pCO2 according to our material.

Conclusion

Concluding, our studies indicate that if tc-pCO2 monitoring is used as a screening method to exclude fetal acidosis, 50% of all fetuses would need further evaluation by fetal scalp blood sampling. This implies that in high risk cases - and at least following a pathological CTG - tc-pCO2 monitoring needs to be supplementet by tissue-pH monitoring in about half of the patients, the only alternative being repeated scalp blood sampling.

References

(1) Nickelsen C, SG Thomsen, T Weber: Eur J Obstet Gynecol Reprod Biol 22 (1986) 215
(2) Severinghaus JW, M Stafford, AN Thonstroem: Acta Anaesth Scand (Suppl 68) (1978) 9
(3) Nickelsen C, T Weber: J Perinat Med (in press)
(4) Nickelsen C, T Weber: Br J Obstet Gynecol 93 (1986) 1268
(5) Nickelsen C, T Weber: Br J Obstet Gynecol 93 (1986) 1272

LACTATE IN THE HUMAN FETUS

M. Katz, E. Lunenfeld, I. Meizner, M. Mazor, B. Piura

Department of Obstetrics and Gynecology, Soroka University Hospital, Faculty of Health Sciences, Ben-Gurion University of the Negev, Beer-Sheva, Israel

Introduction

Lactic acid or α -hydroxyproprionic acid is an organic acid which belongs to the family of carboxylic acids. Lactic acid is found in juices of certain plants and in soil. In the human, lactate is produced by the skeletal muscle, skin, blood cells, brain and eye tissues during anaerobic glucolysis. Lactic acid was first isolated by a Swedish chemist, Carl Wilhelm Scheele, in 1780. In its pure form lactic acid is a colorless, crystaline substance, which melts at 18°C and is highly hydrophilic absorbing rapidly moisture from the atmosphere. The interest with lactate metabolism in the mother and fetus begins in the late twenties with the work published by Bell and Cunningham in the British Journal of Medicine, 1928 (1). The paper is called "The metabolism and acidity of fetal tissues and fluids". The authors found that umbilical cord blood lactate is twice as high as maternal venous. Three years later, in 1931, Eastman and McLane (2) reported that lactate values in umbilical cord at delivery are higher than in the fetus. They explain this rise by "lactate infusion" from the mother in cases of normal infants. As for cases with high lactate they believe that it is of endogenous production due to fetal asphyxia.

What is remarkable that their conclusions are mostly correct after more than 50 years and endless investigations. The formation of excessive amounts of lactic acid in response to acute metabolic demands in the face of temporarily inadequate tissue oxygen is a commonly recognized phenomenon. For example, during vigorous exercise there is an increase in muscular demand for oxygen and due to the oxygen deficit the energy requirement is supplemented by anaerobic metabolism of glucogen. The release of energy is then accompanied by a rise in formation of lactic acid. Such source of energy is quite inefficient in terms of caloric production since for each gram molecule of lactic acid produced the free amount of energy is about ten times less than by the oxidation of the corresponding amount of lactic acid to carbon dioxide and water (3). But in a time of need, this is an extremely important mean of energy production which enables the organism to function, without harm, for brief periods of time in the absence of oxygen. To this forum, the capability to utilise anaerobic metabolism as a source of energy is of particular interest. We are dealing with an area in which our patient, the fetus, appears to be deprived physiologically of his normally low oxygen supply at frequent intervals during labor and delivery, and where, due to a multitude of pathologic processes, the fetal well-being may both depend as well as be jeopardized, by anaerobic metabolism and its by-products. The ability to produce lactate begins very early in fetal life, and Villee (4) in 1954 found evidence of lactate production in fetal tissues of seven weeks' gestation. The capability to breakdown glycogen to lactic acid in absence of oxygen was proven by Himwich et al (5) to be a protective measure that enables the immature fetus to survive temporary lack of oxygen. He placed a newborn rat in nitrogen and found that it survived more than expected and its lactate levels were high. After an injection of sodium fluoride or hypoglycemia induced by insulin, survival time was short and the lactate rise minimal.

In his book on "Fetal and Neonatal Hypoxia" Saling concludes - "It is not oxygen but adequate sources of energy which are essential for cell survival. The fetus needs energy to maintain biochemical reactions and osmotic equilibrium" (6).

Before we proceed to discuss the specifics of lactate metabolism in the mother and fetus, please allow me a few physiologic considerations. Metabolically production of lactate is accompanied by the generation of an equivalent number of protons that are released into the body fluids. Those protons which are titrated by bicarbonate and non-bicarbonate body buffers, acidify the intracellular and extracellular environments. By contrast, metabolic removal of lactate consumes an equivalent number of hydrogen ions and thus restores the body's alkali reserve (Fig. 1).

$$CH_3COCOD^- + NADH + H^+ \ (P)$$

$$\rightleftharpoons \quad \text{LACTATE DEHYDROGENASE}$$

$$CH_3CH(DH)COD^- + NAD^+ \ (L)$$

This reversible reaction occurs in the cytosol and is catalysed by the enzyme lactate dehydrogenase (3). Lactate is formed when pyruvate reacts with reduced nicotinamide adenine dinucleotide and is converted back to pyruvate by reactions with the oxidized counterpart of the dinucleotide. Lactate is a metabolic end product and his only metabolic fate is oxidation back to pyruvate.

The intracellular (cytosolic) concentration of lactate is determined by three variables - concentration of pyruvate - produced mainly by anaerobic glycolysis; the ratio between reduced and oxidized nicotinamide adenine dinucleotide - which is also referred as redox (reduction/oxidation) state and the intracellular hydrogen ion concentration.

Lactic acidosis is defined as an acid base disorder in which accumulation of lactic acid reflects the disruption of normal balance between production and utilization. Metabolic acidosis may be caused by two mechanisms, as shown in Fig. 2.

I) PYRUVATE + $DPNH_2 \underset{}{\overset{LDH}{\rightleftharpoons}}$ LACTATE + DPN

II) LACTATE = [PYRUVATE] X K $\frac{[DPNH_2]}{[DPN]}$

MECHANISM	CAUSE	L/P RATIO
A. INCREASED PYRUVATE	HYPOCAPNIA INFUSIONS OF BICARBONATE GLUCOSE & INSULIN CATECHOLAMINE	UNCHANGED
B. ALTERATIONS OXIDATION DPN DUE TO TISSUE OXYGEN DEBT	HYPOXEMIA CIRCULATORY FAILURE	INCREASED

The first, which is essentially benign, results from an increase in pyruvate concentration with a parallel rise in lactate concentration and thus no change of the lactate/pyruvate ratio. Increase in pyruvate was found in response to hyperventilation and hypocapnia, alkalosis induced by infusion of bicarbonate, infusion of glucose and insulin and rise in catecholamines - on withdrawal of the stimulus pyruvate and lactate quickly will return to their normal values.

The second mechanism which is caused by alteration of oxygenation, leads to a rise in lactate without a corresponding rise in pyruvate - changing thereby the lactate-pyruvate ratio in proportion to oxygen debt. In the human fetus lactic acidemia is a result of inadequate oxygen supply (6).

Fig. 3 taken from Saling's (6) book, summarizes the events that lead to fetal metabolic acidosis.

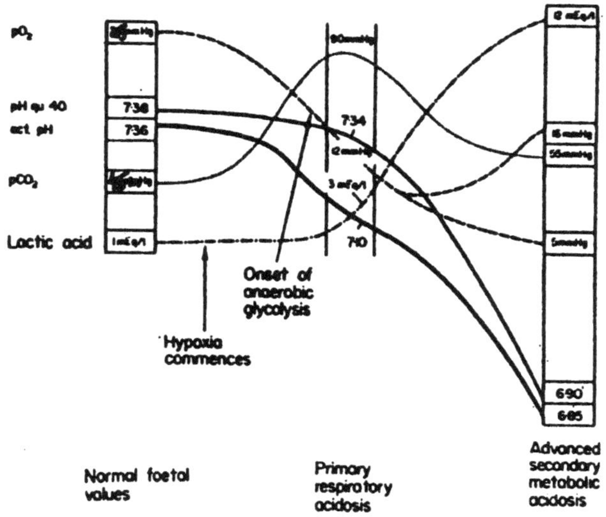

One has to keep in mind that a decrease in oxygen tension in the fetus even when small, may cause a shift of the oxygen dissociation curve, leading to a marked decrease of tissue oxygen saturation and content, and to excessive accumulation of lactic acid. The fetus has only limited capability to protect itself from high lactate levels, because fetal kidneys excrete fixed acids very slowly and the transfer to the mother is limited. Liver, renal cortex, heart and placenta are all lactate-consuming organs. They can use lactate - via pyruvate - as a substance for gluconeogenesis and oxidize it to CO_2 and water - provided the necessary amount of oxygen is available (3). In a study published in 1981 Myers et al (7) reported that in fetal monkeys, even though the primary cause of tissue injury was oxygen deprivation it was the degree of accumulation of lactic acid that determined the extent and severity of brain edema and necrosis (Fig. 4).

In those cases, if death does not result from brainstem compression or the development of cardiogenic shock shortly after resuscitation, survival with lifelong disability can be expected.

What are the normal acid-base characteristics of mother and fetus and how do they change in labor?

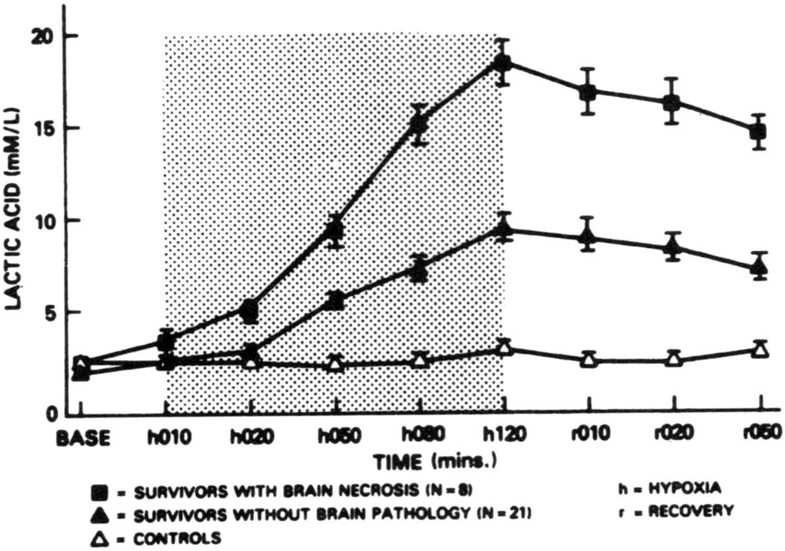

Low et al (8) in a paper published in the Am. J. Obstet. Gyn. in 1974 described the maternal and fetal acid-base, lactate and pyruvate characteristics during labor and delivery in 140 normal patients. Analysing maternal venous blood they found that there is a small decrease of buffer base with a twofold increase in lactate during the labor. The increase in lactate and decrease in pH occur at delivery (Tab. 1).

TABLE 1. The Acid-base, Lactate, and Pyruvate Concentrations in Maternal Venous Blood at the Onset of Labor, Middle of Labor, Second Stage, and Delivery.

	Onset of labor (No. = 28)		Middle of labor (No. = 33)		Second Stage (No. = 98)		Delivery (No. = 40)	
	Mean	S.D.	Mean	S.D.	Mean	S.D.	Mean	S.D.
pH	7.408	0.03	7.433	0.05	7.423	0.06	7.	0.05
Pco_2(mm.Hg)	32.4	3.0	31.3	5.0	30.0	5.0	33.2	5.6
Buffer base (mEq./L.)	42.2	1.7	43.3	1.6	42.2	1.7	41.3	1.7
Lactate								
mmoles/L.	1.36	0.37	1.50	0.52	2.34	1.22	2.89	1.30
mg.%	9.9	2.7	10.8	3.7	16.7	8.5	20.7	9.5
Pyruvate								
mmoles/L.	0.14	0.03	0.14	0.03	0.20	0.08	0.22	0.08
mg.%	0.98	0.21	0.99	0.24	1.4	0.57	1.56	0.57
Lactate/pyruvate ratio	10.0		10.6		11.7		13.4	

In the normal fetus these data refer only to cord values at delivery, but this proves clearly that umbilical artery lactate is higher than this in umbilical vein (Tab. 2).

The twofold increase in lactate concentration in the normal fetus, with a parallel increase in the lactate-pyruvate ratio indicates a minor degree of tissue oxygen debt in the fetus. Low's data were thereafter confirmed by extensive work of Dellenbach (9), Smith (10) and many others.

One may, therefore, conclude that minor acid base changes occur during normal delivery and lead to a rise in lactate levels with a consequent drop

TABLE 2. The Acid-base Characteristics in Fetal Capillary Blood One Hour Prior to Delivery and the Acid-base, Lactate, and Pyruvate Concentrations in Umbilical Vein and Artery Blood at Delivery

	Late first stage (No. = 10)		Delivery - vein (No. = 140)		Delivery-artery (No. = 133)	
	Mean	S.D.	Mean	S.D.	Mean	S.D.
pH	7.313	0.05	7.340	0.05	7.270	0.05
PCO_2 (mm.Hg.)	45.0	7.0	39.6	5.5	50.7	6.8
Buffer base (mEq./L.)	42.2	2.0	42.8	2.0	41.1	2.5
Lactate						
mmoles/L.			2.81	1.18	3.29	1.39
mg.%			19.4	8.1	22.7	9.6
Pyruv{te						
mmoles/L.			0.18	0.05	0.19	0.05
mg.%			1.2	0.36	1.3	0.35
Lactate/pyruvate ratio			16.0		17.0	

in pH in both mother and fetus. Dellenbach et al. (11) followed the acid base changes and lactate concentration in arterial and venous blood of 60 patignts, at term, during elective Cesarean section. In each case they obtained simultaneously samples from maternal iliac artery, uterine vein, antecubital vein, umbilical artery and umbilical vein. What they found is that the level of maternal lactate is identical regardless of the sampling site. The gradient of lactate was always positive between fetus and mother and umbilical artery and umbilical vein, indicating that the human fetus produces lactic acid and that a part of lactate disappears when it crosses the placenta (Fig. 5).

Schneider et al investigated the influence of type of anesthesia used for elective Cesarean sections on lactic acid concentration in mother and fetus in 22 patients with general and 9 with epidural anesthesia. The first blood sample was taken 15 minutes prior to anesthesia, then the second at the delivery of the newborn (Fig. 6).

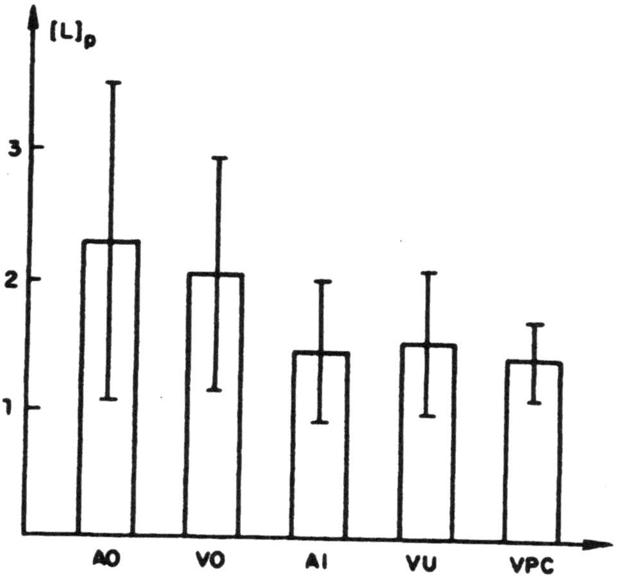
[L]p
3
2
1
AO
VO
AI
VU
VPC

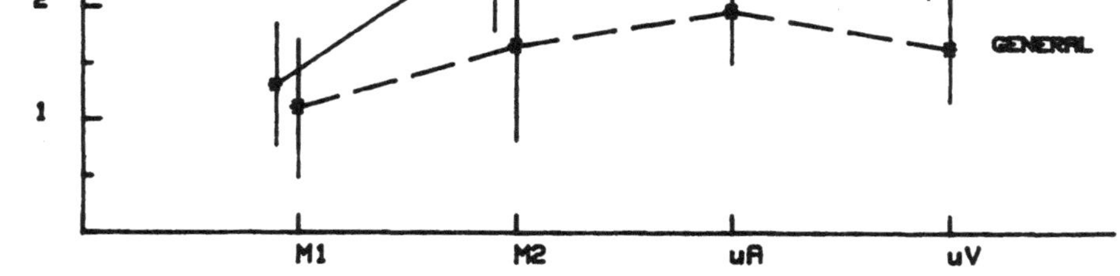
mM/1
LACTATE (mM/1)
3
2
1
EPIDURAL
GENERAL
M1
M2
uA
uV

Lactate levels in mother rose in both types of anesthesia, most probably during induction time, but the increase was more significant in those with epidural than with general anesthesia.

One can only speculate that the possible explanation for this rise would be an increased lactate production due to temporary tissue hypoxia and stimulation of lactate metabolism as a result of stress or anxiety. In their study umbilical artery lactate and vein lactate were higher than maternal which shows once more that without labor, under a steady state the fetus produces lactate, and because of placental permeability a slow but constant flow of lactate from the fetus to the mother follows.

Moll (13) studied the accumulation and disappearance of lactate in the fetus of a guinea pig who also has a hemochorial placenta and according to him where fetal oxygenation is optimal placental transfer and fetal utilization of lactate are almost equal. Otey et al (14) suggested that the placenta serves as a buffer for the fetus. Low (15) in 1979 states that based on his work the changes of lactate and pyruvate that occur in mother and fetus during labor are parallel but independent. He based this statement on the fact that maternal lactate in normal and "complicated" pregnancies was quite similar whereas the "complicated" group had a much higher fetal lactate level than the normal.

Lactic acid is present in high concentration in amniotic fluid - Raiha (16) believes that this high concentration is a result of fetal excretion and probably due to glycolysis. High activity of lactic dehydrogenase was found in amniotic fluid by Lapin and Freeman (17) (Fig. 7).

In summary, based on human observations and animal studies, it seems that little, if any, lactate and pyruvate are crossing the placenta. If transplacental transfer exists it will be by diffusion and it is, therefore, logical that the movement will be from the fetus to the mother.

Increase in lactate in fetus and mother, most probably occurs independently. We know now that maternal lactate rises during labor and delivery and the question is what is the cause of this rise and at which stage of labor does it happen.

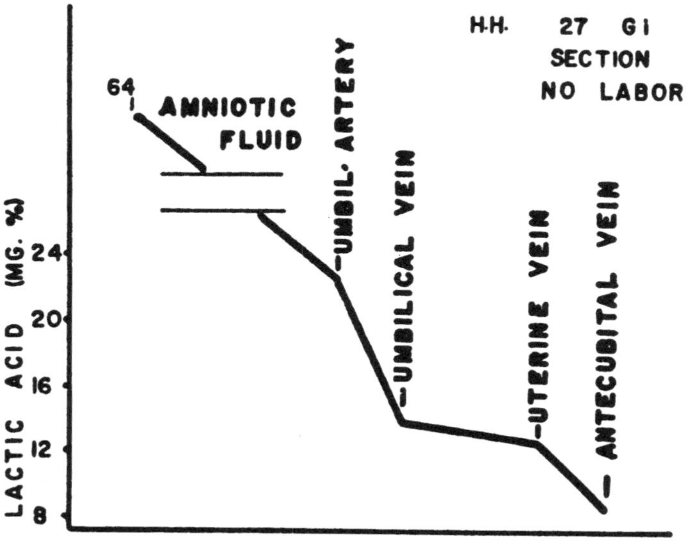

Hendricks (18) found that there is a gradual increase of lactate during active labor with a peak level at time of delivery (Fig. 8).

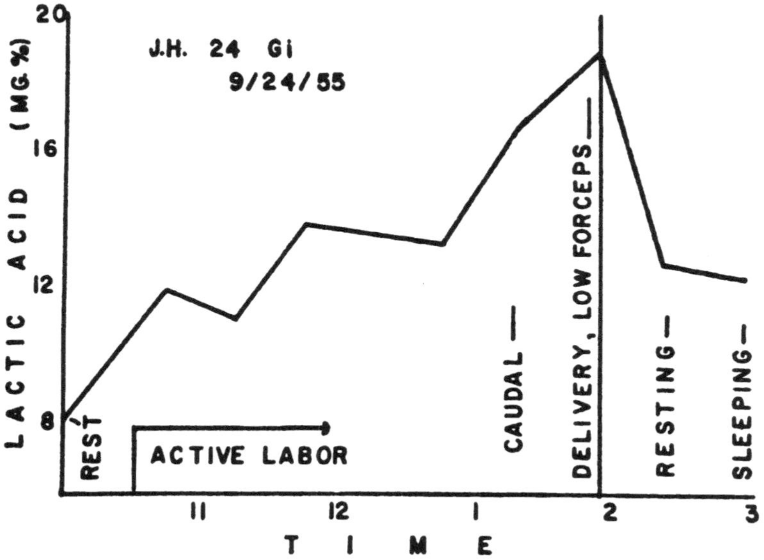

According to Hendricks it may be assumed that at least a major portion of the progressive rise in lactic acid concentration is on the basis of activity of the uterus and/or its contents.

If Hendrick's conclusion is correct, it should point to a state similar to what one can see during exercise when muscular work leads to oxygen utilization greater than supply and as a result, to excessive lactate accumulation.

In order to assess the energy expenditure in normal labor we did the following:
25 healthy parturients were attached by a mouth piece to a metabolic cart which measured every 10 min. for 5 mins. duration, oxygen consumption, CO_2 production, heart rate and respiration rate. At cervical dilatation of 3,6,8 and 10 cm, venous blood samples were obtained for lactate and pH. The mean results of 17 patients are presented (19). (Fig. 9).

MATERNAL METABOLIC PROFILE IN RELATION STAGES OF LABOR AND DELIVERY(mean values)

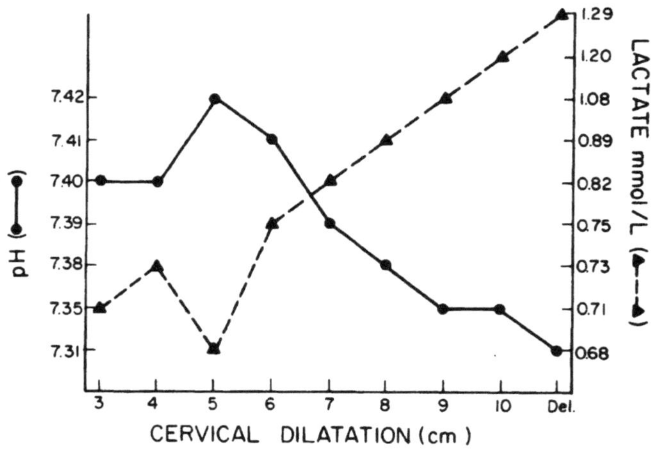

KATZ M., KROL D. et al

Oxygen consumption seems to double during contraction, but returns to precontraction levels in about 30 sec. Maternal glucose levels remained stable throughout labor. The pH dropped by 0.05 pH units and the lactate levels were almost stable until the second stage of labor, during which the rise was in a range of 40-50%.

Based on our data we tend to believe that the major contributor to the rise in maternal lactate is not only the uterus but also maternal skeletal and abdominal muscles, participating in the process of delivery.

In a prospective study of 254 patients who had a vaginal delivery of a singleton fetus, we found that the mean maternal venous lactate levels during latent phase was 0.85 ± 0.14 mmol/L, and rose at delivery up to 2.14 ± 0.28 (range from 1.34 - 5.40). The mean umbilical artery lactate was 2.87 and umbilical vein 2.31 mmol/L (20).

When Haberey et al (21) compared maternal and fetal lactate levels in labor, they found an almost linear correlation between those two, throughout labor and delivery in normal cases. Maternal values remained persistently lower also in those defined as prepathological and pathological cases in which fetal lactate rose significantly - thus once more providing proof that fetal metabolic acidosis during labor and delivery is very unlikely to be secondary to lactate produced by mother (Fig. 10).

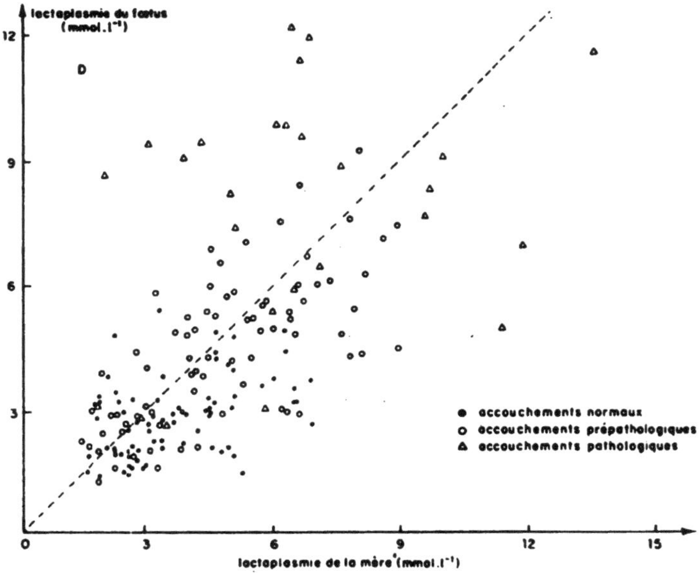

When lactate levels assessed in capillary scalp blood smaples were related to fetal heart rate patterns it was shown by Young (22), Smith (10) and Katz (20) that a high correlation exists between cardiotocographic indicators of fetal asphyxia and hyperlacticemia (Fig. 11).

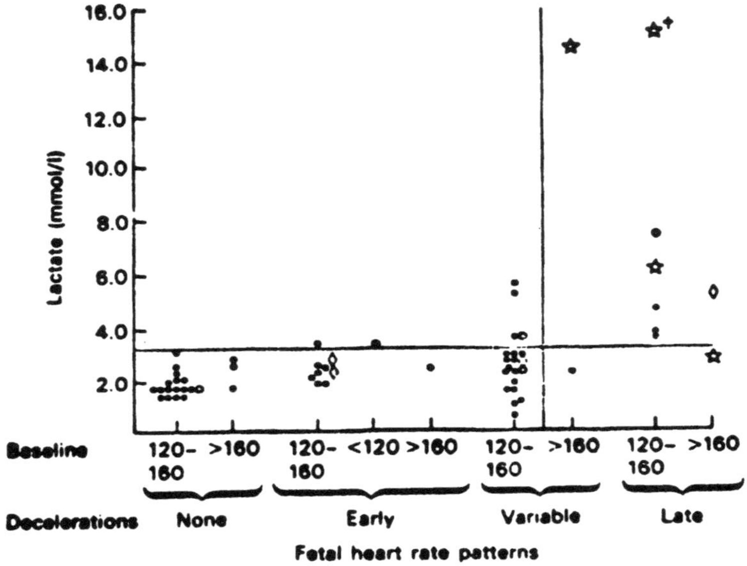

We then looked upon the relation between meconium stained amniotic fluid and lactate levels. The results were interesting but not surprising - lactate in umbilical artery and vein was in the normal range when light meconium was seen.

In the 22 patients (out of 254) who had thick meconium, lactate was 4.15 ± 1.2 mmol/L in the umbilical artery and 2.76 ± 1.27 in umbilical vein. The difference in lactate levels in the two groups of meconium was statistically significant (p 0.01). This finding supports the view that thick meconium is indeed a sign of fetal hypoxia (23).

There is one more subject, quite controversial, which we would like to address, and it is that of duration of second stage of labor - and its impact on neonatal well-being. The second stage is characterized by uterine contractions that are both frequent and prolonged. During those contractions there is a marked reduction in placental perfusion.

Beard and Morris (24) and many other investigators found a decrease in base excess and fall in scalp capillary pH during second stage, and Wood et al (25) had shown that prolongation of expulsion period is associated with maternal and fetal acidosis. Out of 254 cases in our study we had accurate data on duration of second stage in 148 patients (20).

In 101 patients in whom second stage lasted from 1 to 75 minutes maternal lactate levels were ascertained, showing a rise in values which were statistically not significant.

The changes with duration of second stage were significant in umbilical artery and umbilical vein (Tab. 3).

TABLE 3. Umbilical and Maternal Lactate (mmol/l) by Duration of the Second Stage of Labor and Parity

	Duration of second stage (min)			
Blood sample	1-15	16-30	> 30	P*
Umbilical artery				
Primiparae	2.4 (1.7-4.2) (n = 18)	2.9 (1.0-5.5) (n = 18)	3.1 (1.8-6.5) (n = 26)	<0.025
Multiparae	2.4 (0.8-5.2) (n = 54)	2.6 (1.6-4.2) (n = 17)	2.9 (1.5-9.8) (n = 10)	<0.023
Umbilical vein				
Primiparae	2.6 (1.3-3.5) (n = 21)	2.7 (1.4-4.8) (n = 19)	3.2 (1.6-7.2) (n = 27)	<0.015
Multiparae	2.2 (0.8-4.6) (n = 54)	2.8 (1.5-5.7) (n = 17)	2.9 (1.5-2.9) (n = 10)	<0.013
Maternal vein				
Primiparae	3.1 (2.1-4.3) (n = 18)	3.5 (2.5-7.4) (n = 10)	3.5 (1.7-6.5) (n = 21)	NS
Multiparae	3.0 (1.3-6.7) (n = 40)	3.4 (1.8-5.4) (n = 9)	4.0 (3.7-4.4) (n = 3)	NS

Results are medians (range), n is the number of samples
*Statistical analysis used Kruskal-Wallis one way ANOVA.

Although in this study the changes in pO_2 and pCO_2 were less marked than those in pH and lactate we know from the work of Huch et al and Pearson that during second stage there is a decline in oxygen supply to the fetus leading to a mild respiratory acidosis of the fetus which resolves quickly after delivery. It is therefore important to avoid excessive prolongation of second stage of labor during which lactic acid accumulation and metabolic acidosis may develop.

Studies done by Smith (10), Low (8) and Young (22),as well as our own prove that lactic acid measurements are as good predictors of neonatal outcome as scalp pH. The availability of a quick assessment using micro samples of scalp blood should enable us to diagnose the development of oxygen deficit maybe even before significant drop in scalp pH. It is our belief that lactate measurements in labor in the fetus and mother should be added to the armamentarium of means of surveillance in labor and delivery.

References

(1) Bell WB, I Cunningham, M Jowett: The metabolism and acidity of the foetal tissues and fluids. Br Med J 1 (1928) 126

(2) Eastman NJ, CM McLane: Foetal blood studies. II The lactic acid content of umbilical cord blood under various conditions. Bull Johns Hopkins Hosp 48 (1931) 261

(3) Madias NE: Lactic acidosis. Kidney International 29 (1986) 752

(4) Villee CA: In: Reynolds SRM (ed.): The intermediary metabolism of human fetal tissues. Symposia on quantitative biology. 19 (1954) 186

(5) Himwich HE et al as quoted in: Hendricks CH: Studies on lactic acid metabolism in pregnancy and labor. Am J Obst Gynecol 73 (1957) 492

(6) Saling E: Foetal and neonatal hypoxia. E Arnold Ltd., London 1967

(7) Myers RE, KR Wagner, G DeCourten: Lactic acid accumulation in tissue as the cause of brain injury and death in cardiogenic shock from asphyxia. In: Lauersen NH, HM Hochberg (eds): Clinical Perinatal Monitoring. Williams and Wilkins, Baltimore 1981

(8) Low JA, SR Pancham, D Worthington, RW Boston: Acid-base, lactate and pyruvate characteristics of the normal obstetric patient and fetus during the intrapartum period. Am J Obstet Gynecol 120 (1974) 862

(9) Dellenbach P, F Piquard, RR Hsuing et al: Lactaplasmie maternelle et foetale au cours de l'accouchement. Rev Fr Gynecol Obstet 12 (1981) 841

(10) Smith NC, WP Soutter, F Sharp et al: Fetal scalp blood lactate as an indicator of intrapartum hypoxia. Brit J Obstet Gynecol 90 (1983) 821

(11) Dellenbach P, F Piquard, R Hsuing et al: Lactaplasmie maternelle et foetale dans 60 cas de cesarienne prophylactique. Rev Fr Gynecol Obstet 12 (1981) 831

(12) Schneider H, R Huch, A Huch et al: The influence of anesthesia for Cesarean section on lactic acid concentration in maternal and fetal blood. Abstracts of the 7th European Congress of Perinatal Medicine. Barcelona (1980) 120
(13) Moll W, E Kastendieck: Accumulation and disappearance of lactate in a fetus with a hemochorial placenta. The role of placental transfer and fetal metabolism. J Perinat Med 2 (1978) 246
(14) Otey E, V Stenger, D Eitzman, H Prystowsky: Further observation on the relationships of pyruvate and lactate in human pregnancy. Am J Obst Gynecol 97 (1967) 1076
(15) Low JA, SR Pancham, WN Piercy et al: Maternal and fetal lactate characteristics during labor and delivery. In: Bossart H, C Perret (eds.): "Lactate in acute conditions". Karger, Basel 1979
(16) Raiha NCR: Organic acids in fetal blood and amniotic fluid. Pediatrics 17 (1963) 1025
(17) Lupin R, MM Freeman: Enzymes in amniotic fluid and maternal serum. Am J Obstet Gynecol 83 (1962) 1337
(18) Hendricks CH: Studies in lactic acid metabolism in pregnancy and labor. Am J Obstet Gynecol 73 (1957) 492
(19) Katz M, D Kroll, I Shapiro et al: Energy expenditure in normal labor. (In preparation)
(20) Katz M, E Lunenfeld, I Meizner et al: The effect of the duration of the second stage of labor on the acid-base state of the fetus. Brit J Obstet Gynaecol 94 (1987) 425
(21) Haberey P, F Piquard, R Hsuing et al: Etude critique de l'acidose transmise. Rev Fr Gynecol Obstet 76 (1981) 877
(22) Suidan JS, BK Young: Acidosis in the vigorous newborn. Obstet Gynecol 65 (1985) 361
(23) Katz M, E Lunenfeld, I Meizner: Umbilical blood lactate in patients with meconium stained amniotic fluid. (In preparation)
(24) Beard RW, ED Morris, SG Clayton: -pH of foetal capillary blood as an indicator of the condition of the foetus. J Obstet Gynaecol Br Commonw 74 (1967) 812
(25) Wood C, KH Ng, D Hounslow: Time - an important variable in normal delivery. J Obstet Gynaecol Br Commonw 80 (1973) 295

HUMAN RESEARCH ON LACTATE

S. Schmidt

Department of Obstetrics & Gynecology, University of Bonn,
Sigmund-Freud-Str. 25, D-5300 Bonn, FRG

The accumulation of lactate acid in the brain in association with hypoxia causes edema and tissue necrosis (2,5,6). Current methods of detecting intrapartu lactate acid accumulation are not entirely satisfactory. As has been shown the intracellular lactate acid accumulation in the brain tissue can be approximately estimated by detection of changes of lactate concentration in the fetal blood. In this way a detection of changes of lactate acid concentration in the fetal blood should be a precise indicator of the degree of fetal stress during labour (1,7).

During a clinical trial we evaluated the question to what extend it is possible to estimate the lactate in the fetal blood by measuring other biochemical parameters.

Method

This investigation was performed in 125 high-risk-deliveries where lactate acid was measured by means of an encymatic test (Boehringer). Samples were either collected using the fetal blood sample-technique by Saling or by sampling fetal blood from the umbilical artery at the moment of delivery. Additionally capillary blood samples were collected from the mother. The synchroneously collected data were compared by using the linear correlation analysis, the sensitivity, the specifity, the negativ predictive value and the positive predictive value.

The parameters compared were the P_{O_2}, P_{CO_2}, BE, pH and the PH qu 40. Furthermore the linear correlation between the difference of the fetal and maternal BE and the lactat in the fetal blood was calculated (4).

Results

As the mean value of lactate concentration in the samples of fetal blood collected during delivery (FBA) we calculated 2.96$\pm$ 1.51 mmol/l. The value of the samples from the umbilical artery (UA) was significantly higher (2a = 0.05). Here we found a value of 3.87$\pm$1.78 mmol/l. While maternal values collected during labour were not statistically different from fetal values, fetal values exceeded the maternal values at the moment of delivery (Fig. 1). Comparing the values of the lactate concentration in the fetal blood with the other biochemical parameters we found in most items a statistically significant correlation, but though due to the amount of scattering of the values the correlation coefficients were low (<0,5) Fig. 2 - 6). An overview of our statistical evaluation is given on table 1 (tab. 1). For the P_{CO_2} and P_{O_2} we did not find a significant correlation between these value and lactate acid concentration in the fetal blood - collected from the umbilical artery. The sensitifity, the specifity, the positive predictive and the negative predictive value were calculated. Comparing the data of the fetal blood we used a cut off point for the lactat concentrations of 3 mmol/l, P_{CO_2} 55 mmHg, P_{O_2} 15 mmHg, BE 6 mmol/l, pH 7.25, pH qu 40 7.25.

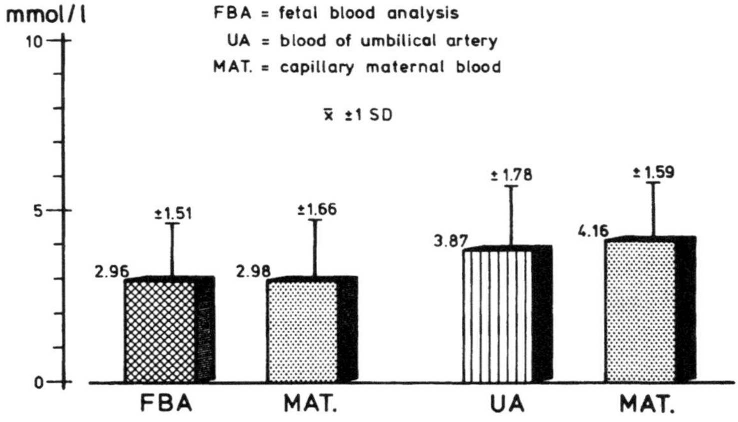

Fig. 1 Mean value (x) and standard deviation (SD) of the lactate concentration (mmol/l) in synchroneously collected scamples of maternal and fetal blood.

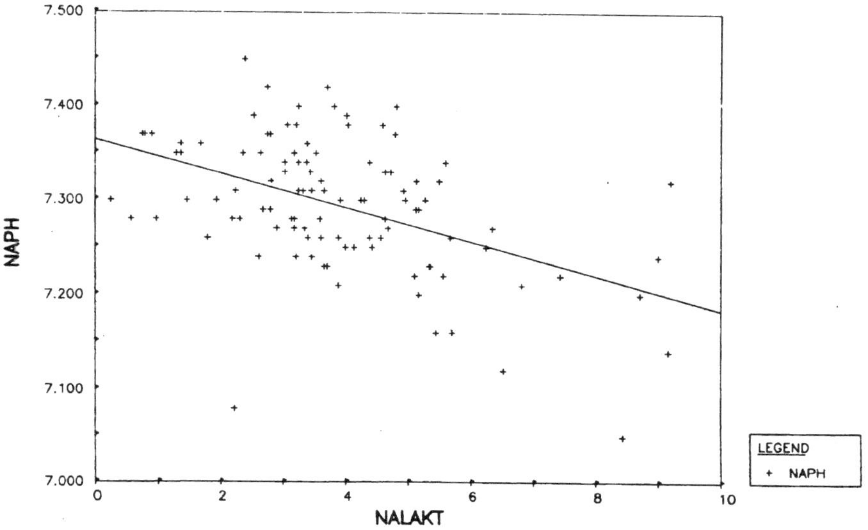

Fig. 2 Correlation between the lactate concentration (mmol/l) and the pH in blood samples from the umbilical artery (UA).

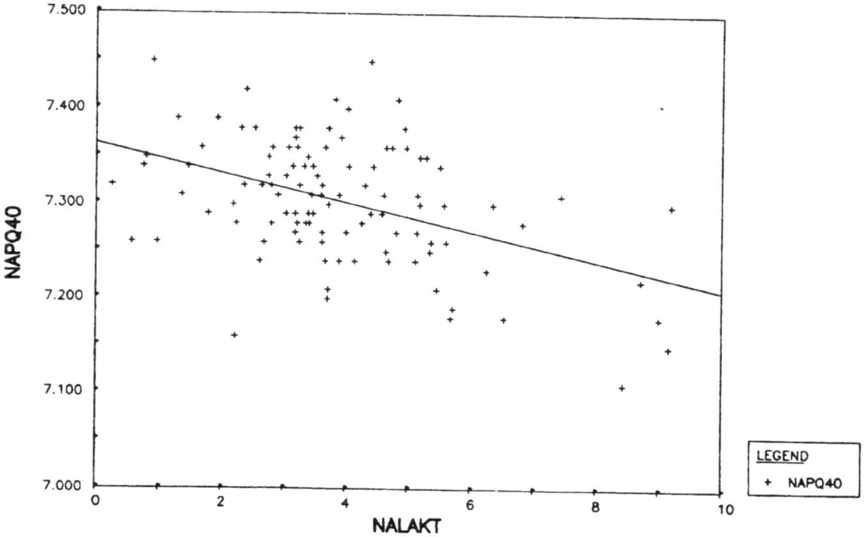

Fig. 3 Correlation between the lactate concentration (mmol/l) and the pH in blood samples from the fetus after equillibration at a P_{CO_2} of 40 mmHg.

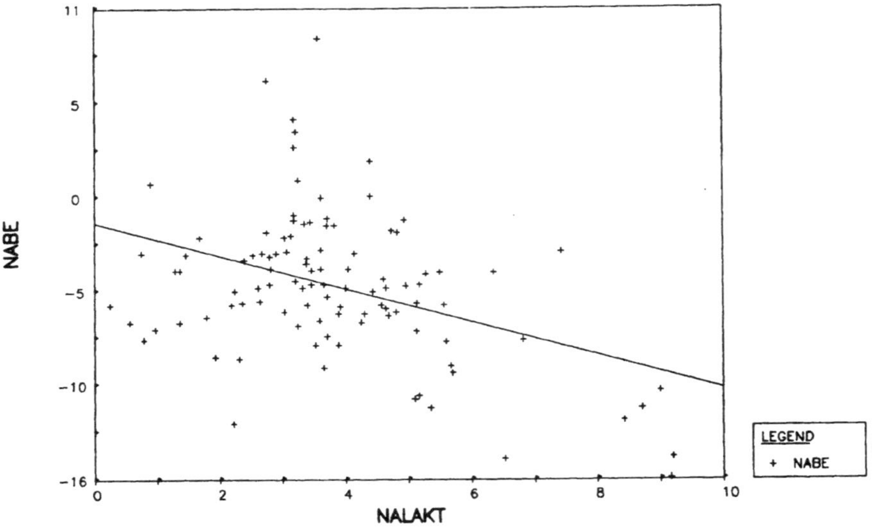

Fig. 4 Correlation between the lactate concentration (mmol/l) and the base excess (BE) in scamples of fetal blood.

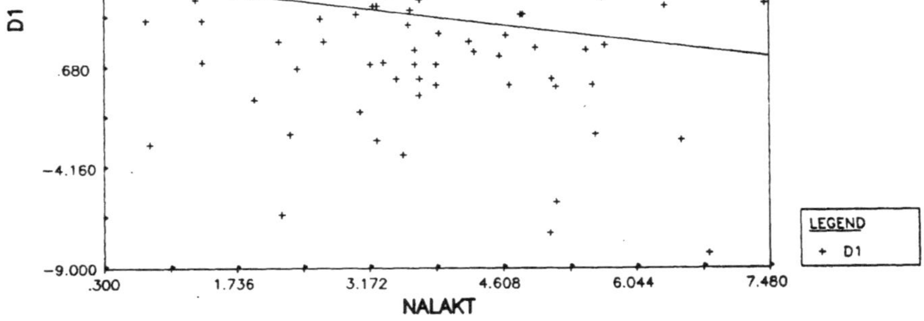

Fig. 5 Correlation between the lactate concentration (mmol/l) and the difference between the fetal and maternal base excess (BE) = D1 (mmol/l).

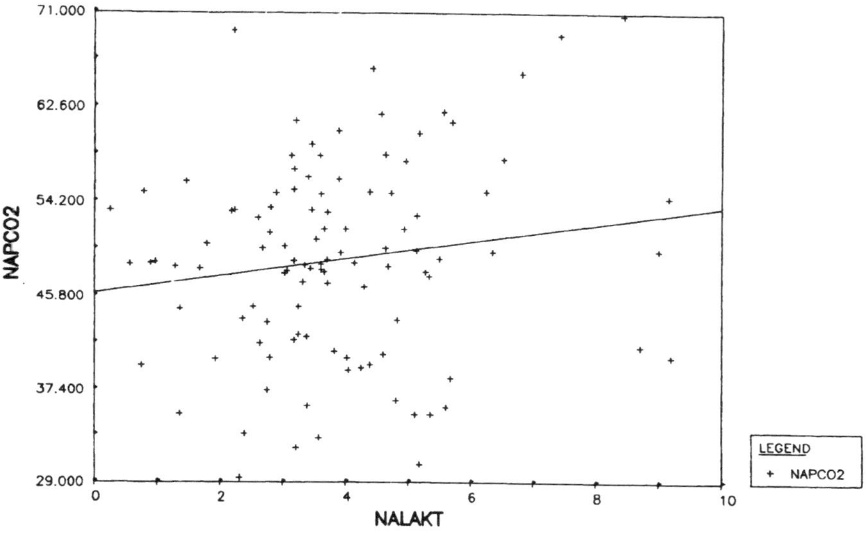

Fig. 6 Correlation between lactate concentration (mmol/l) and P_{CO_2} (mmHg) in samples from the umbilical artery.

Tab. 1 Result of the analysis of the linear correlation (p,r) the positive (ppv) and negative (npv) predictive value, the sensitifity and specificity to detect lactate accumulation (> 3 mmol/l).

	p	r	ppv	npv	sens.	spec.	n	
pH	< 0,00001	- 0,46	92%	34%	31%	93%	108	
pHqu 4o	< 0,00001	- 0,43	90%	3o%	22%	93%	107	
BE	< 0,00001	- 0,40	76%	3o%	41%	65%	104	UA
Diff BE fet-BEmat	< 0,01	- 0,26	31%	71%	87%	14%	101	
P_{CO_2}	> 0,05	- 0,15	90%	31%	23%	93%	107	
P_{O_2}	> 0,05	- 0,12	85%	34%	4o%	82%	101	
pH	≤ 0,01	- 0,36	57%	63%	21%	90%	46	
pHqu 4o	≤ 0,01	- 0,49	100%	61%	24%	100%	45	
BE	≤ 0,01	- 0,45	56%	78%	5o%	82%	34	FBA
Diff BE fet-BE mat	> 0,05	- 0,22	28%	6o%	56%	32%	31	
P_{CO_2}	> 0,05	- 0,07	60%	59%	3o%	83%	38	
P_{O_2}	< 0,01	- 0,44	55%	68%	46%	75%	34	

The results of this calculation is presented in table 1. The highest value for the positive predictive value was calculated for the pH (92%) when considering the values measured in the umbilical artery. The negative predictive value though was calculated to be <50% for all investigated biochemical parameters. The highest value for the specificity during labour was found for the pH qu 40 (93%). The result when calculating the sensitifity was disappointing for all parameters. The best result was achieved by using the difference between fetal and maternal values (87% respectively 56%) for values during labour respectively at the moment of delivery.

Comment

The measurement of lactate concentrations in blood samples from the fetus is still time consuming and cumbersome. Its potential value has been well demonstrated in animal experiments (5).
It is potential to predict the result of the clinical assessment of the newborn has also been approved (7). As the results of this paper implicated there is only limited value of other single parameters to detect lactate concentration of above 3 mmol/l.
The fact that gas values (P_{O2} and P_{CO2}) do not correlate with lactate concentrations can be expected from the pathophysiology of acute intrauterine complications as with proceeding lactate accumulation during centralisation of the circulation P_{O2} might rise again due to the O_2-cunsumption being reduced. The results also demonstrate that materno-fetal blood analysis have a potential in the diagnosis of fetal lactate accumulation (4). Further development though should aim at the development of techniques to measure lactate directly and in a less time consuming way during routine surveillance of the fetus.

References

(1) Bretscher J, E Saling: pH values in the human fetus during labour. Am J Obstet Gynecol 97 (1967) 906
(2) Hendricks CH: Studies on lactic acid metabolism in pregnancy and labour. Am J Obstet Gynecol 73 (1957) 492
(3) Hsiung R, F Piquard, A Schaefer, J Machu, P Haberey, P Dellenbach: Lactaplasmie maternelle et foetale au cours de l'accouchement. II Accouchement Pathologiques. Rev Fr Gyneécol Obstét 76 (1981) 853

(4) Kastendieck E, G Yilmar, A Jensen, G Horner: Die fetomaternale Blutanalyse (FBMA) zur Diagnose der Hypoxie des Feten sub partu. Z Geburtsh u Perinat 190 (1986) 14
(5) Myers RE, KR Wagner, GD Courten: Lactic acid accumulation in tissue as cause of brain injury and death in cardiogenic shock from asphyxia. In: Lauersen NH, HM Hochberg (eds.) Clinical perinatal biochemical monitoring. Williams & Wilkins, Baltimore 1981
(6) Niswander KR: In: Pitkin RM, FJ Zlatnik (eds.): The year book of obstetrics and gynecology. Asphyxia in the fetus and cerebral palsy. Year Book Medical Publishers Inc., Chicago 1983
(7) Suidan JS: outcome of fetuses with lactic acidemia. Am J Obstet Gynecol 150 (1984) 33

THE RELATIONSHIP BETWEEN ARTERIAL AND TISSUE PO_2 IN THE FETAL LAMB[1]

Molly E. Towell

Department of Obstetrics & Gynecology, McMaster University
Hamilton, Ontario L8N 3Z5

The relationship between arterial and tissue PO_2 is not well understood in the adult, let alone in the fetus. Figure 1 shows the pathway for oxygen through the maternal lungs and pulmonary circulation to the systemic circulation. For the fetus, there is an additional step of transfer across the placenta to fetal blood, and thence via the fetal heart to systemic circulation and fetal tissues. It should also be noted that well oxygenated blood from the placenta is mixed with deoxygenated blood in the fetal circulation before it is distributed to fetal tissues thus further reducing the concentration of oxygen in fetal blood circulating to tissues. It can be assumed that both in mother and fetus there will be a marked drop in PO_2 between arterial blood and tissues as oxygen diffuses to the oxygen consuming sites in the mitochondria. This cascade of oxygen is illustrated diagramatically in the lower part of Figure 1. The major difference which emerges between mother and fetus is the low PO_2 of fetal blood compared with maternal blood. This is likely to impose an even lower tissue PO_2 on the fetus than that found in the adult and values reported for fetal tissues have ranged from 1 to 20 mmHg (1-6).

Our studies have been carried out in fetal sheep and we have been measuring both blood and tissue PO_2. The questions that we have posed are as follows:

1. What are the absolute values for tissue PO_2 in the fetal lamb?
2. What is the correlation between blood and tissue PO_2?
3. What factors can affect this correlation such as increasing gestational age and duration of implantation of electrodes, and how does hypoxemia and asphyxia affect tissue PO_2?
4. What are the absolute values for PO_2 in the newborn lamb?

[1] Supported by a grant from the Ontario Heart and Stroke Foundation, Canada.

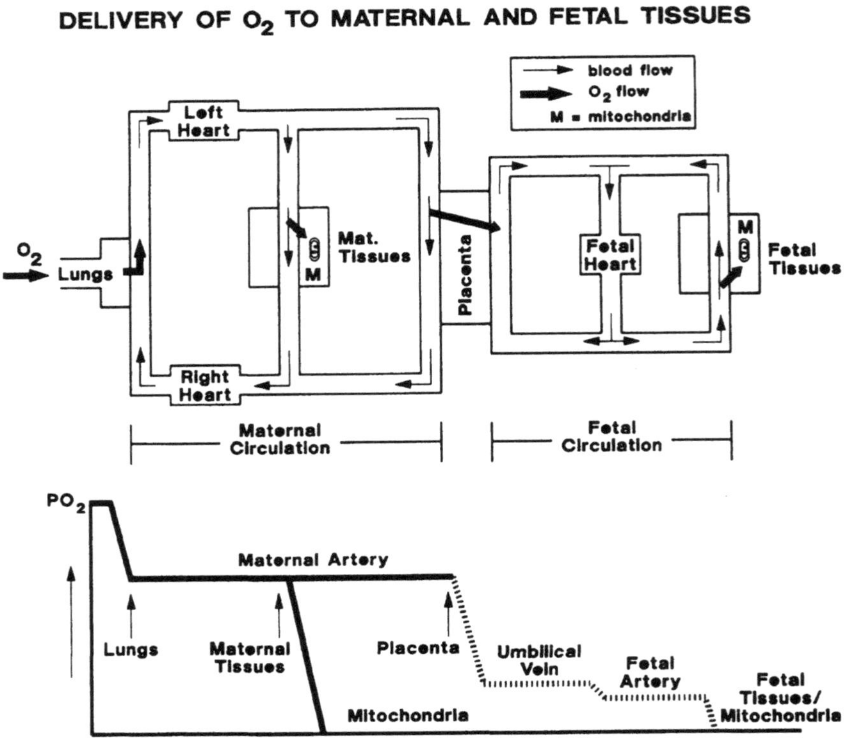

Figure 1

Upper: The pathway for oxygen can be traced via maternal lungs, left heart and systemic circulation to maternal tissues. For the fetus, there is an additional step of transfer across the placenta and thence via fetal heart to systemic circulation and fetal tissues.

Lower: Illustrates the cascade of oxygen from air via maternal lungs to maternal arterial blood and tissues. Note the sharp drop in $P0_2$ as oxygen diffuses from blood to maternal tissues and mitochondria. There is also a sharp drop in $P0_2$ across the placenta and a further drop takes place as oxygen diffuses from fetal blood to fetal tissues and mitochondria.

Electrodes Used to Measure Oxygen Tension

The electrodes we have used have been both intravascular and chronically implanted tissue PO_2 electrodes. The intravascular PO_2 sensor is a commercially available polarographic electrode mounted in the tip of a double-lumen catheter (Venus Oxygen Probe - Orange

Medical Instruments Ltd., High Wycombe, England). It is a Clark-type electrode and is difficult to maintain for long periods of time in chronic fetal sheep preparations because heparinization of fetal blood has to be continuously maintained.

The tissue PO_2 sensor is a custom-made galvanic electrode made available to us through the courtesy of Professor S. P. Bessman, University of Southern California at Los Angeles. This is a fairly large electrode measuring 3 mm which is housed in an acrylic disc of 1 cm diameter (Figure 2). Unlike the Clark electrode, the galvanic electrode does not require a polarization current placed across the anode-cathode pair, i.e., it is a self-generating $P0_2$ electrode from which current or voltage can be measured directly (7). The electrode is placed within tissue layers, e.g. subcutaneous tissue, or on the surface of muscle or dura mater overlying cerebral cortex, and we believe that it measures tissue fluid $P0_2$. This method represents a different approach to the measurement of tissue P02 and cannot be compared with measurements by needle electrodes introduced in a blind fashion into different locations within the tissue, both intracellular and extracellular. It is comparable with the Clark type heated transcutaneous electrode (8) with respect to its size and the area of tissue to which it is applied. However, the galvanic electrode is not heated and measurements represent actual readings obtained at the temperature of the tissue, i.e. about 39-40°C in the fetal lamb.

After removal of the electrode from subcutaneous tissues, one can see a smooth pocket of tissue which surrounds the electrode and is separated from it by a thin layer of tissue fluid. Figure 2 shows the appearance of the dura overlying cerebral cortex in a newborn lamb after reflecting the galvanic O_2 electrode which had been applied before birth.

Results

Typical recordings from a fetal lamb in which a dural PO_2 electrode had been implanted are shown in Figure 3. Note that tissue PO_2 is extremely low, with a baseline around 4 mmHg. Note also the repetitive dips in PO_2 which are characteristic of a normally functioning electrode and a fetal lamb in good condition. The dips in tissue PO_2 appear to be associated with bursts of uterine electromyographic activity which represent uterine contractions. Episodes of mild tachycardia are also associated with the dips in PO_2, as we have previously reported (9).

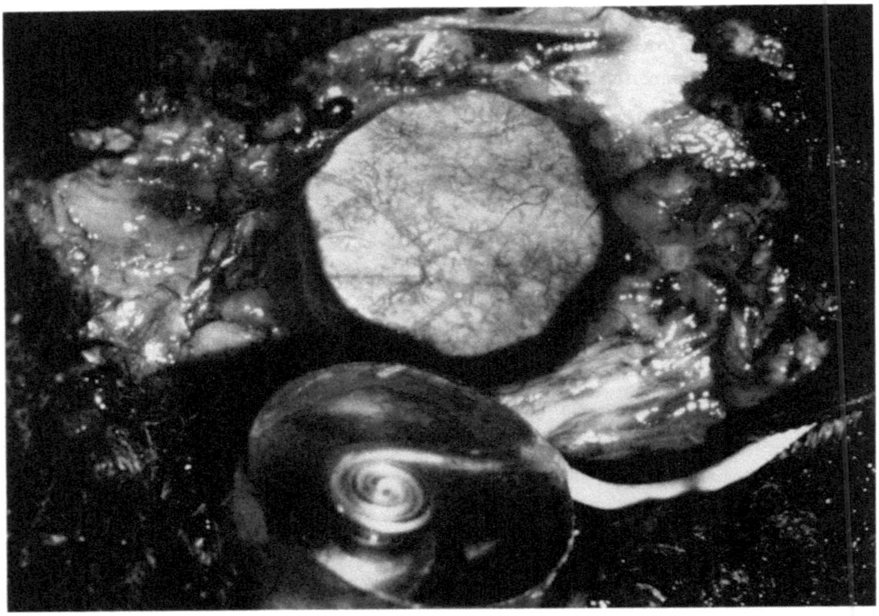

Figure 2

Galvanic PO_2 electrode reflected from its site of implantation on the dura overlying cerebral cortex in a newborn lamb aged 5 days. The electrode had been implanted 9 days before birth. Diameter of burr hole in skull and acrylic disc housing PO_2 electrode is 1 cm.

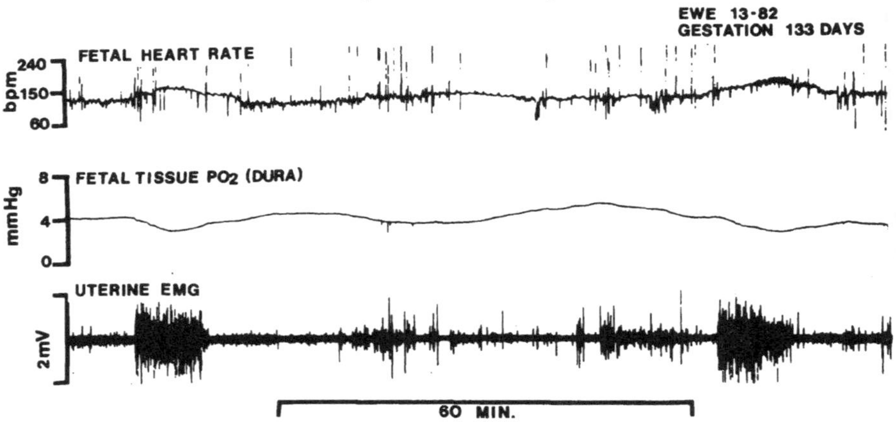

Figure 3

Simultaneous recording of tissue (dura) PO_2 and heart rate in a fetal lamb at 133 days gestation. Electromyographic (EMG) activity recorded from uterine wall.

Relationship between blood and tissue PO_2 under physiologic conditions

Simultaneous recordings of fetal arterial and tissue PO_2 have been examined in the fetal lamb. Figure 4 shows the computerized output from a recording of arterial blood and tissue PO_2 in a fetal lamb at 142 days gestation; the lamb was delivered in good condition 2-3 days after this recording was made. Frequent dips in PO_2 can be seen and it should be noted that tissue PO_2 faithfully reproduced the dips seen in arterial blood. Note that arterial PO_2 ranged from 17 to 22 mm Hg while tissue (subcutaneous) PO_2 ranged from 4 to 6 mmHg, i.e. a ratio of approximately 4:1.

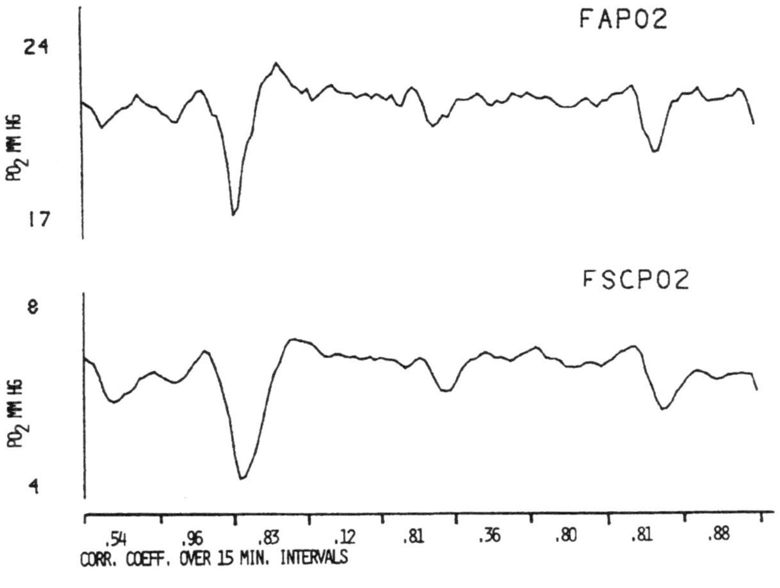

Figure 4

Computer output plot of 135 minutes recording of arterial PO_2 ($FAPO_2$) and subcutaneous tissue PO_2 ($FSCPO_2$) in a fetal lamb at 142 days gestation (term = 147 days). Data averaged over 30s intervals . Intravascular and tissue electrode implanted at 105 days gestation. Note the correlation coefficient (r) values below for arterial vs tissue PO_2 over 15 minute intervals.

In order to document the relationship between arterial and tissue PO_2 in more detail, the correlation coefficient (r) between these two variables was examined over 15 minute intervals. The r values are shown below the recording in Figure 4. The correlation coefficient was generally high with r values greater than or equal to .80. On the other hand, correlation was less significant when there was little deviation or no dips in PO_2. This is not unexpected since correlation requires deviation in values to show significance and the r value will be zero if two straight lines are correlated.

Mean fetal arterial PO_2 was measured over many days from the time of implantation of electrodes in five pregnant ewes up to the time of delivery. This interval ranged from 8-40 days. All lambs were born in good condition at or near term. Figure 5 shows mean values of PO_2 representing 6-30 hours of recording at various intervals from implantation of electrodes. Arterial blood PO_2 remained relatively stable up to term. Tissue PO_2, however, showed a sharp decline from the time of implantation of electrodes and did not stabilize until about 10-15 days later.

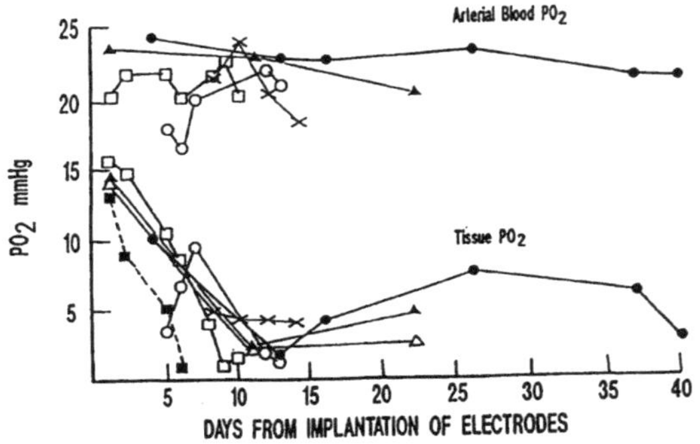

Figure 5

Mean fetal arterial and tissue PO_2 in 5 fetal lambs from the time of electrode implantation (105-129 days gestation) until delivery or electrode failure. Each point represents mean value for 6 - 30 hours of data. ×, △, ○, ■, ●, represent subcutaneous tissue PO_2 electrodes in 5 fetal lambs and ▲, □, represent dural PO_2 electrodes in 2 of the 5 fetuses.

The mean correlation coefficient (r) between arterial and tissue PO_2 plotted against elapsed time from implantation of electrodes and gestational age (days from delivery) is shown in Figure 6. Correlation improved with increasing time from implantation and with increasing gestational age. It is not clear at the present time which factors, i.e. increasing time from implantation of electrodes or increasing fetal maturity, had the most important influence on the relationship between arterial and tissue PO_2. However, it is clear that it improved with time. This may reflect the development of a good micro-circulation around the electrode.

Alternatively, increasing fetal maturity with more deviation in oxygen tension (dips in PO_2) due to increased uterine activity, may have heightened the relationship between blood and tissue PO_2.

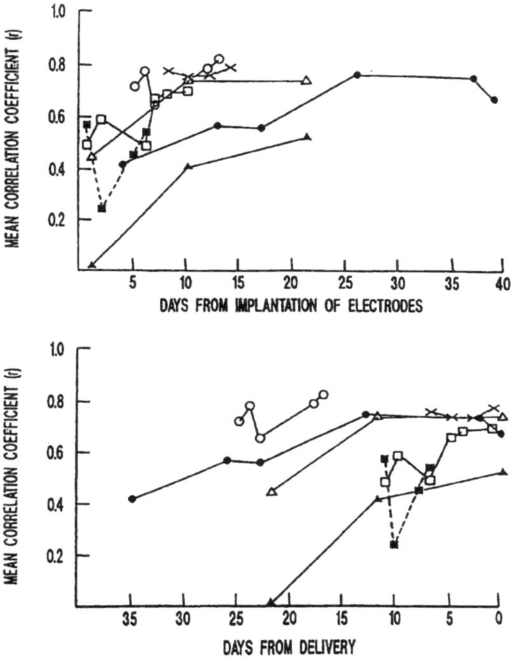

Figure 6

Effect of elapsed time from implantation of electrodes (above) and increasing fetal maturity (below) on mean correlation coefficient (r) between arterial blood and tissue PO_2 in 5 fetal lambs. Each point represents mean r values for 8 - 60 periods of 30 minutes each. Note the trend towards higher r values with increasing time from implantation of electrodes. ×, △, ○, ■, ●, represent subcutaneous tissue PO_2 electrodes and ▲, □, represent dural PO_2 electrodes in 2 of the 5 fetuses.

Relationship between blood and tissue PO_2 under pathological conditions

Maternal hypoxemia was studied by administering 10% O_2 to the pregnant ewe. Figure 7 shows a recording of maternal tissue PO_2 from the surface of the uterus and fetal tissue PO_2 from subcutaneous tissue and the surface of fetal muscle. It can be seen that maternal tissue

PO_2 returned quite rapidly towards baseline values, whereas fetal tissue PO_2 returned slowly following the period of hypoxemia. The delay in reoxygenation of fetal tissues may be due in part to the extra step in oxygen transfer across the placenta and in part to the admixture of well oxygenated umbilical venous blood with deoxygenated blood before distribution to fetal tissues.

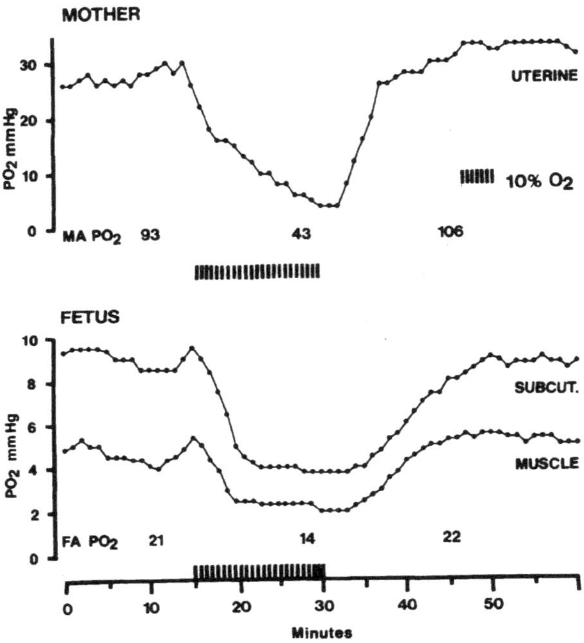

Figure 7

Effect of administration of 10% 0_2 to a pregnant ewe, on maternal tissue $P0_2$ (uterine wall) and fetal tissue $P0_2$ (subcutaneous and muscle). Note the slow return to baseline tissue $P0_2$ values in the fetus compared with the mother. Intermittent blood samples obtained from maternal carotid artery ($MAP0_2$) and fetal carotid artery ($FAP0_2$).

We have also used the model of umbilical cord compression as a means of studying fetal hypoxia. Figure 8 shows the results of an experiment in which fetal arterial blood PO_2 and tissue PO_2 were examined simultaneously during a moderate degree of umbilical cord compression for 30 minutes; arterial pH fell from 7.36 to 7.27 during this period. Note that fetal arterial PO_2 initially fell rapidly but began to increase again during compression although pH continued to fall. The increase in blood PO_2 can probably be attributed in part to a shift to the right in the fetal oxygen dissociation curve due to the development of acidosis.

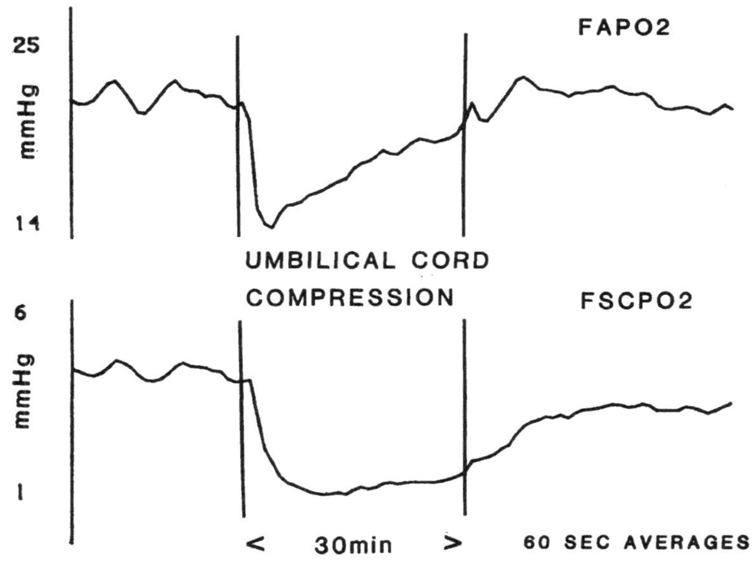

Figure 8

Computer outplot of fetal arterial PO_2 ($FAPO_2$) during a typical experiment in which the umbilical cord was partially compressed for 30 minutes. The correlation coefficient (r) for the control (pre-compression) period was 0.77 and for each successive 30 minute period was -.15, .39 and .90. Thus correlation between blood and tissue PO_2 was poor during compression and the initial 30 minutes of the recovery period.

Despite the rise in blood PO_2, subcutaneous tissue PO_2 remained depressed throughout the period of cord compression. When the cord was released, tissue PO_2 increased slowly in comparison with arterial PO_2, which was rapidly restored to pre-compression values. Although the explanation for this phenomenon is not yet clear, it can be postulated that the failure of tissue PO_2 to reflect blood PO_2 may depend on factors which alter blood flow to the tissue, e.g. peripheral vasoconstriction due to catecholamine release.

Tissue PO_2 in the newborn lamb

We have also had an opportunity to measure newborn tissue PO_2 following delivery of fetal lambs with implanted PO_2 electrodes. Figure 9 shows the record from a newborn lamb in which PO_2 electrodes were implanted approximately 10 days before delivery. Note that at one day of age, muscle and subcutaneous tissue PO_2 had risen to values 3-5 times those found in the fetus, i.e. to 15-35 mm Hg compared with from levels of < 5 mm Hg before birth.

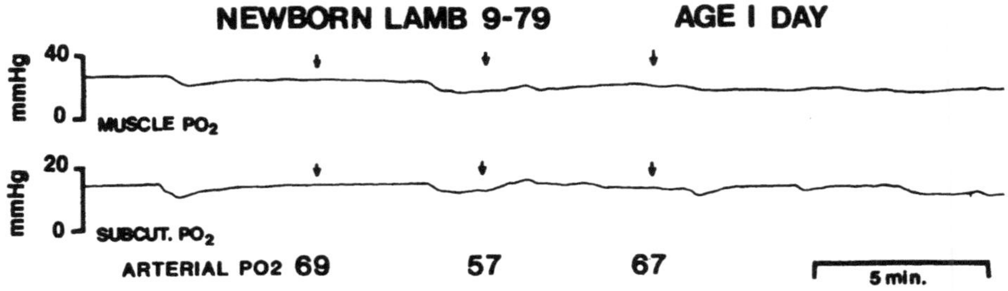

Figure 9

Muscle and subcutaneous tissue PO_2 recorded in a newborn lamb aged 1 day. Galvanic tissue electrodes implanted in the fetus before birth. Carotid arterial blood samples obtained at points indicated by arrows for measurement of PO_2 in vitro.

Intermittent dips of tissue PO_2 were again seen, as in fetal PO_2 recordings, and these appeared to correlate with arterial PO_2 levels measured in vitro. The nature and cause of these dips is not clear at the present time.

Conclusions

1. Absolute values of tissue PO_2 in the fetal lamb are generally <10 mm Hg and frequently <5 mm Hg.
2. Tissue PO_2 increases in the newborn lamb, as anticipated, after birth.
3. There is a high degree of correlation (0.75 or better) between fetal arterial and tissue PO_2 under the following conditions: (i) normal physiologic; (ii) tissue electrodes implanted for at least 7-14 days; (iii) increasing fetal maturity.

4. Correlation between fetal arterial blood and tissue PO_2 is heightened during PO_2 dips, which occur under normal physiologic conditions in the fetal lamb, and with increasing frequency as term is approached.
5. Fetal tissue PO_2 remains depressed after maternal hypoxemia and after fetal asphyxia induced by umbilical cord compression. Recovery to baseline is slow in fetal tissue compared with fetal arterial blood. Thus it is possible that tissue PO_2 may provide us with a better indication of fetal status than blood PO_2 under conditions of hypoxemia or asphyxia.

Acknowledgements

Expert technical assistance from G. Madhavan, J. Johnson and T. Dinh and typing assistance from J. Bennett and J. Paci is gratefully acknowledged.

References

(1) Erdmann W: In: Longo LD, H Bartels (eds.): Respiratory gas exchange and blood flow in the placenta. DHEW Pub No (NIH) 73-361 Bethesda 1973
(2) Staisch KJ, B Nuwayhid, RO Bauer, L Welsh, CR Brinkmann: Obstet Gynecol 47 (1976) 587
(3) Guilbeau EJ, DD Reneau: Microvascular Res 13 (1977) 241
(4) Aarnoudse JG, B Oeseburg, G Kwant, HJ Huisjes, WG Zijlstra: Biol Neonate 38 (1980) 49
(5) Towell ME, I Regier, I Lysak, D Sayler SP Bessmann: In: Bicher HI, DF Bruley, eds: Oxygen transport to tissue-IV. Plenum Pub Corp, New York, NY (1983) 37
(6) Towell ME, J Johnson, I Lysak, DF Sayler, SP Bessman: Biochem Med 33 (1985) 180
(7) Bessman SP, RD Schultz: Trans Amer Soc Artif Int Organs 19 (1973) 361
(8) Huch A, R Huch, B Arner, G Rooth: Scand J Clin Lab Invest 31 (1973) 269
(9) Towell ME, J Johnson, G Madhavan, H de Bruin: In: Bruley D, HI Bicher, D Reneau (eds.): Oxygen transport to tissue-VI. Plenum Pub Corp, New York 1985

TISSUE pH/pCO2 AND CONTINUOUS BASE EXCESS MONITORING IN THE HUMAN FETUS

T. Weber

Department of Obstetrics and Gynecology, Hvidovre Hospital, University of Copenhagen, Denmark

C. Nickelsen

Department og Obstetrics and Gynecology, Rigshospitalet, University of Copenhagen, Denmark

Introduction

During the last three decades intrapartum fetal mortality has decreased all over the western world. In most clinics this decrease in fetal mortality rate has been paralleled by an increased frequency of electronic monitoring of the fetus during labor. However, even large randomized trials comparing electronic monitoring of the fetus to a group of fetuses not being monitored have failed to prove a beneficial effect of electronic monitoring concerning the perinatal mortality. When major neurological handicaps are evaluated in the same series even this condition have not been influenced by electronic monitoring in the few randomized trials (1). These results may be explained by the few intrapartum fetal deaths and the few neurologically damaged fetuses in both groups. However, it stresses the need for other ways of fetal monitoring.

As the ultimate goal of fetal monitoring is to prevent cell damage of the most vital and most sensitive organs (e.g. brain and heart), a method of fetal monitoring which detects a decreased oxygen/energy supply to these organs before cell damage occur is necessary. If the exchange of oxygen and carbon dioxide between the maternal and fetal circulation is diminished (e.g. cord compression, placental insufficiency, hypertone of the uterus) the first change will be a decreased pO2 and increased pCO2. By definition this is a respiratory acidosis and this condition has been proved to be without deleterious effect to the fetus as long as the oxygen level is sufficient to maintain normal metabolism. However, if the oxygen level decreases further, the metabolism changes from aerobic to anaerobic pass-ways causing accumulation of organic acids and especially lactic acid. In this case the acidosis is changing from a respiratory to a metabolic acidosis (or a combination of the two types of acidosis). Further, in animal experiments it has been shown that metabolic acidosis caused by hypoxia parallels the degree of brain damage (2).

As a consequence of these pathophysiological changes during fetal hypoxia measurement of the fetal acid base state seems to be the best way of assessing fetal well being. Measurement of pH is a good indicator of acidosis, but it is not possible to evaluate the degree of metabolic/respiratory components if only the pH is known.

Monitoring of the pCO2 might be a good indicator of a beginning acidosis, but if pH is not known many cases of slight respiratory acidosis - which do not need intervention - might be classified as pathological. Consequently, the ideal would be to monitor both the pH and the pCO2 simultaneously and continuously.

In the following the results of tissue pH monitoring during labor, transcutaneous pCO2 monitoring during labor, and combined tissue pH and transcutaneous pCO2 monitoring during labor will be described.

Tissue pH (tpH) monitoring during labor

At present only one electrode has been used for tissue pH monitoring during labor. This electrode (Roche) is a combined glass- and reference electrode which is applied to the fetal head using a special application tool making it possible to apply the electrode without the use of an amnioscope. The electrode is held into position by a spiral electrode, the tip of the glass electrode being situated in the subcutaneous tissue. The pH is displayed on a pH-meter and on the cardiotocogram as a continuous line or dots every ten seconds. In 229 consecutive tpH monitorings in which the tissue pH was monitored until delivery the tissue pH correlated very well to the umbilical artery blood pH ($r = 0.71$). Tissue pH values between 7.02 and 7.40 were seen in the serie. All monitorings were performed by the two authors.

The duration of monitoring in all 337 cases was very long in most cases and more than 20 % were monitored 300 - 500 minutes. Most patients were monitored between two and five hours and only 59 patients were monitored for less than 30 minutes. The drift of the electrode did not depend on the duration of monitoring. Sixty-seven per cent of the monitorings were successful, 10% were partly successful (a stable tracing was obtained but the tissue pH was not stable until the delivery), and 23% of the tracings were unsuccessful with no stable tissue pH value obtained. After the first 150 monitorings in which the tissue pH value did not influence the management of labor, the following management of labor was established:

1. In case of severe bradycardia ($<$ 70 beats per minute) obstetrical intervention was performed.
2. In all other cases obstetrical intervention was only performed if tissue pH was $<$ 7.20 (7.15 if delivery could be expected within 15 minutes or if t-pH increased within 15 minutes).
3. A pathological CTG was treated conservatively (e.g. by oxygen, changing of maternal position or by i.v. NaCl)

Seventy-two patients were managed by t-pH. In these patients we found a significant reduction of vacuum extraction/outlet forceps deliveries compared to a matched group of patients in which the pH was not used in the management of labor (25.8 versus 8.6%, p = 0.007). The state of the neonates did not differ between the two groups (3).

Transcutaneous pCO2 monitoring during labor

The transcutaneous pCO2 electrode can be applied to the fetal head with a suction or a glue fixation ring. No difference between simultaneously obtained values from a glue fixated electrode and a suction fixated electrode was found (4).

Within the EEC (European Economic Community) a multicenter trial was set up. In this trial all patients were monitored by a Radiometer electrode heated to 41°C. The study was performed by the authors from Denmark, by Stephan Schmidt and Erich Saling from Berlin, John Spencer and Paul Johnson from Oxford, and Martin Bergmans and Herman van Geijn from Amsterdam. The number of patients were 39, 31, 50, 14 from the four mentioned centers. The correlation between the umbilical artery blood pCO2 and the transcutaneous pCO2 (tc-pCO2) obtained 0-10 minutes before delivery was acceptable, (n = 49, r = 0.49), but this correlation was not as good at the correlation found by the authors in an earlier study in which an electrode temperature of 44°C was used (r = 0.77, n = 64). The correlation between the arterial umbilical artery blood pCO2 and transcutaneous pCO2 was best in the centers that were used to tc-pCO2 monitoring.

In three acidotic neonates (arterial umbilical artery blood pH less than 7.15) tc-pCO2 was monitored 0 - 10 minutes before delivery. The tc-pCO2 was increased in one case (13.3 kPa), but it was normal in the other two cases (7.5 and 5.1 kPa).

Especially during the last part of labor pCO2 may change rather rapidly. Nevertheless, comparing the tc-pCO2 value obtained until 0-60 minutes before delivery gives an impression of the value of the method as applied by the centers involved. Therefore, we looked at the possibility of predicting neonatal acidosis from the transcutaneous pCO2 value 0-60 minutes before delivery. The best discrimination was obtained by a pCO2 limit of 8.0 kPa, but even then only four out of ten acidotic neonates were found, the six false negatives having tc-pCO2 values evenly distributed between 5 and 8 kPa. Further, 31/104 of the neonates with umbilical artery blood pH above 7.15 had a transcutaneous pCO2 value above 8.0.

Consequently, the detection rate was only 40%. An increased tc-pCO2 was found in 30% of the normal neonates.

If tc-pCO2 was normal, the risk of neonatal acidosis was 6/79 = 8% - i.e. almost the same as in the total material (risk 10/114 = 9%). This means that in the EEC-material a low tc-pCO2 value 0-60 minutes and even 0-10 minutes before delivery was not reassuring concerning the acid base state of the newborn.

The umbilical artery blood pCO2 and the last transcutaneous pCO2 value at the different centers was studied. In most centers the mean umbilical artery blood pCO2 was the same (6.6 - 6.7 kPa), one center having a mean umbilical artery blood pCO2 of 7.1. In contrast the tc-pCO2 varied between the centers with mean values from 6.8 to 8.0 kPa. The highest mean values were found at the two centers with the highest experience in tc-pCO2 monitoring. Theoretically, the metabolic production of CO2 of the outer skin layer should contribute to the tc- pCO2 with 0.5 kPa and the tc-pCO2 should consequently be 0.5 kPa higher than the umbilical artery pCO2. This was nearly the case in the two most experienced departments.

The success rates of tc-pCO2 monitoring was quite different between the centers. In the most experienced center the success rate was close to 100% in the first state of labor but in one of the less experienced centers the success rate was only 75% in the first stage. In the second stage the highest success rate was 75% and the lowest only 25%.

The average number of applications during the first stage varied between 1.1 and 1.5, whereas the average number of applications during the second stage varied much more (0.1 - 1.2 applications). An increased number of applications did not seem to increase the success rate.

All centers had many cases in which the electrode was applied very early in labor, most applications being performed at a cervical dilatation of 3-4 cm.

Monitoring was performed for more than five hours in 10% of the cases,and only 27% were monitored for less than one hour.

The only complication seen after the monitoring was a small red spot following suction fixation. No burns caused by the heated electrode was found.

In four cases the umbilical artery blood pH was less that 7.10.

In the first case meconium stained liquor was found and Caesarean section was performed because of suspected fetal distress. A child of 2450 gram (40 weeks) was delivered. Apgar scores were 6/1 and 10/5. Umbilical artery blood pH was 7.09 but the pCO2 was not measured in the umbilical cord blood. The child was intubated and ventilated but did not need transport to the pediatric unit. The tc-pCO2 was monitored for four hours but not during the last 30 minutes before delivery. The tc-pCO2 value increased from 6.5 kPa to 13.3 kPa (last value). In this case transcutaneous pCO2 predicted fetal acidosis.

In the next case a child was delivered spontaneously with Apgar 8/1, 9/5. The weight was 3290 gram (40 weeks). Umbilical artery pH was 7.01 (vein 7.10), pCO2 was 11.6 kPa (vein 8.3 kPa), and standard base excess was -9.2 mEq/l (vein -10.1). Artificial ventilation was performed but no intubation was necessary. No transport to pediatric unit. Tc-pCO2 monitoring was performed for almost two hours and until birth. The transcutaneous pCO2 increased from 8.0 to 13.4 kPa during monitoring. In this case acidosis was predicted by an increasing tc-pCO2.

In the third case Caesarean section was performed for suspected fetal distress. Fetal weight was 3000 gram (40 weeks). Apgar scores were 7/1, 9/5. Umbilical artery blood pH 7.09 (vein 7.13) pCO2 8.3 kPa (vein 8.2) - SBE -10.4 mEq/l(vein -6.3). No artificial ventilation was needed and the child did not need transport to pediatric unit. Tc-pCO2 monitoring was performed for 95 minutes but was discontinued one hour before birth. The tc-pCO2 increased from 5.1 to 9.3 kPa. In this case the tc-pCO2 increase was only moderate but the monitoring was not performed for the last hour before birth and might had predicted the acidosis more clearly during the last hour before birth.

The last case of severe neonatal acidosis followed Caesarean section performed for dystocia. Fetal weight was 3660 gram (39 weeks), Apgar scores were 6/1, 9/5. No artificial ventilation was performed and the neonate was not transported to the pediatric unit. pH was 7.08 (vein 7.14) - pCO2 8.0 kPa (vein 7.0) and SBE -11.7 mEq/l(vein -10.2). Tc-pCO2 monitoring was performed for almost 4 hours, but monitoring was discontinued more than one hour before birth. The tc-pCO2 value (5.5 kPa) did not increase during monitoring. In this case the fetal acidosis could not be predicted by transcutaneous pCO2 monitoring, but monitoring was not performed during the last hour before birth. Further, the case was mostly a case of metabolic acidosis as SBE was low and as pCO2 was almost normal.

Concluding: two out of four cases were predicted by transcutaneous pCO2 monitoring. The other two cases were not monitored for the last 60 minutes and fetal acidosis might have been predicted if monitoring had been performed throughout labor.

Continuous base excess monitoring during labor

The technique of continuous base excess monitoring during labor is quite difficult to handle. It is necessary to apply an invasive tissue pH electrode and at the same time a transcutaneous $pCO2$ electrode. The tissue pH value and the $pCO2$ value can be noted on the cardiotocogram every ten seconds (e.g. on the labor- and fetal heart rate tracing). At the same time the SBE can be calculated on line using a microcomputer. Following delivery all calculated standard base excess values can be printed out graphically.

In seven cases continuous standard base excess monitoring was performed preceding delivery of a non-acidotic child with normal Apgar scores. In all cases the standard base excess was slightly increasing or constant during delivery (5).

The correlation between the standard base excess of the umbilical artery blood and the calculated standard base excess (calculated from the tissue and the transcutaneous values) was acceptable ($r = 0.66$, $p < 0.05$, $n = 13$) (6).

In two cases we found continuous standard base excess monitoring of special interest.

In the first case the CTG showed a deep deceleration of the fetal heart rate in the first stage of labor followed by an immediate increasing carbon dioxide tension from 7.1 kPa to 9.2 kPa reaching its maximum after 6 minutes and returning to the starting level after 25 minutes. The tissue pH was decreasing from 7.29 just before the deceleration to a minimum of 7.20 after 25 minutes. During the next 20 minutes the tissue pH increased to 7.25 and this value remained unchanged until delivery two hours later. During the first six minutes this represents a respiratory acidosis, but the continued decrease of pH in spite of restoration of the carbon dioxide level can be explained as a complicating metabolic acidosis. The child was born with Apgar scores of 9/1, 10/5.

The second example was a patient who had variable decelerations of the fetal heart rate during the second stage of labor. This was accompanied by a gradual tissue pH decrease from a value of 7.28 to below 7.20. The electrode was reapplied and as the tissue value was still below 7.20, vacuum extraction was performed. The carbon dioxide tension was constantly 5.3 kPa during the first 30 minutes but increased to 8.2 kPa during the last 15 minutes. This example illustrates the development of a metabolic acidosis and the increasing carbon dioxide tension during the last 15 minutes is probably secondary to the metabolic acidosis. Apgar scores were 7/1, 10/3, 3/5 (caused by aspiration). Later the infant quickly recovered and no neonatal morbidity was found. Umbilical artery blood pH was 7.11 and pCO2 was 8.4 kPa ($44^{0}C$ value), the standard base excess was -9.5 mEq/l.

Possible future strategies for intrapartum monitoring

At present none of the mentioned ways of monitoring are ready for routine use. If transcutaneous pCO2 monitoring becomes easier and future studies show that the sensitivity and specificity of the method becomes better with increased experience (especially decreasing the non-monitored period(s) of the last part of labor), transcutaneous pCO2 monitoring might be applied as a screening method in high risk cases and in cases with pathological CTG. If the tc-pCO2 value becomes pathological further evaluation is needed and in this case an invasive method (e.g. a tissue pH electrode) should be applied. Unfortunately, the present tissue pH electrode can not be used routinely as it is very difficult to handle and is very expensive. If a better tissue pH electrode becomes available (e.g. an improved version of the needle electrode which has shown acceptable performance during animal experiments) (7) the best way of monitoring would consequently be:

1. CTG and tc-pCO2 monitoring in all high risk cases.
2. In cases with pathological CTG- and/or pathological tc-pCO2-monitoring this is supplementet with tissue pH monitoring with a pH electrode.
3. Acute intervention for suspected fetal distress is always incated in cases of metabolic acidosis.
4. The obstetrician might try "conservative" treatment (e.g. oxygen, i.v. fluid, change of maternal position) in cases with respiratory acidosis. This should only be tried if spontaneous delivery is expected and actually takes place after a short while - or if the respiratory acidosis is successfully treated by the "conservative" management.

References

(1) MacDonald D, A Grant, M Sheridan-Pereira, P Boylan, I Chalmers: Am J Obstet Gynecol 152 (1985) 524
(2) Myers RE: Am J Obstet Gynecol 112 (1972) 246
(3) Weber T: Acta Obstet Gynecol Scand 61 (1982) 351
(4) Nickelsen C, T Weber: Brit J Obstet Gynaecol 93 (1986) 1268
(5) Nickelsen C, T Weber: Eur J Obstet Gynecol Reprod Biol 21 (1986) 7
(6) Nickelsen C, SG Thomsen, T Weber: Br J Obstet Gynaecol 92 (1985) 220
(7) Nickelsen C, T Weber, AJ Hansen, A Hansen, T Zeuthen: Int J Gynaecol Obstet 24 (1986) 459

The **Journal of Perinatal Medicine** is a truly international forum covering the whole field of perinatal medicine.

The issues include invited **review articles** providing a coverage of theoretical and practical points of view in a particular field, **original contributions** reporting on new results, particularly from the clinical and experimental areas, **technical notes** describing the characteristics of new instruments of methodological improvements, **short communications** and **letters to the Editors.** Each article is followed by comprehensive summaries in English, French and German.

All contributions submitted for publication are critically reviewed by at least two renowned experts in the field in order to ensure constant high quality of the journal.

The **Journal of Perinatal Medicine** is an essential news source for all those perinatologists who wish to keep abreast of progress in perinatal research.

Abstracted/Indexed in: Automatic Subject Citation Alert (ASCA®), Current Contents/Clinical Practice (CC/CP), ISI/BIOMED®, Science Citation Index (SCI®), SCISEARCH®; Index Medicus, Core Journals.

Bei Fragen zur Produktsicherheit wenden Sie sich bitte an:
If you have any questions regarding product safety,
please contact:

Walter de Gruyter GmbH
Genthiner Straße 13
10785 Berlin
productsafety@degruyterbrill.com